THE POWER OF OUR STORY

# Wounds

# to

# Wisdom

# Author's Note

Dear reader, it is our profound hope that the stories within this anthology, as shared by fellow
Protectors-Veterans and First Responders,
will touch your heart and bring to the forefront the power of solidarity that exists within this community, and the value of support that lies within the heart of these authors.

Each story is a testament to resilience, shared with the hope of inspiring others and reinforcing the message that, no matter the obstacles we face, we are never truly alone.

As you embark on this journey through personal accounts, please be aware that some narratives may evoke strong emotions or trigger memories related to psychological or physiological traumas. The following themes may appear in one or more stories:

―――――――― ∽ ――――――――

Alcohol and Alcoholism
Substance Abuse
Suicide and Suicidal Ideation
Loss and Grief
Physical and child abuse
Sexual harrassment and Abuse
Rape
Sexual Exploitation
Self-harm
Mental Illness
Cancer

―――――――― ∽ ――――――――

Additionally, you may encounter coarse language, graphic depictions of combat or accidents, and terminology that some readers may find objectionable. We encourage you to approach these stories with an open heart and mind, honoring the courage it takes to share such intimate experiences. Thank you for joining us on this journey.

Editor: Natalie June Reilly
Cover Design: Book Cover World
Interior Design: 2Creative Minds
PaperBack ISBN: 979-8-9906481-0-4, Ed.1, 2024
eBook ISBN: 979-8-9906481-1-1 Ed. 1, 2024

## *Dedication to All Our Protectors Who Hold That Line*

*Wounds to Wisdom: Healing Through Veteran and First Responder Narratives is a lifeline for those of us on the front lines, battling not only the external threats faced daily but also the internal wounds that can linger long after the sirens and smoke have faded. More than just stories, "Wounds to Wisdom" is a roadmap for healing. It distinguishes between the wounds that still ache and the scars that serve as reminders of our strength. It's a beacon of hope, guiding us toward the light of shared experience and collective resilience. In these pages, you'll find the stories of our fellow Protectors—Veterans and First Responders—who have faced the darkness head-on and emerged stronger.*

*This book is a testament to the brotherhood and sisterhood that binds us together. It reminds us that no matter how isolated we may feel, suffering in silence, we are never truly alone. Through the voices of our fellow authors, we hear the echoes of our own experiences—reassurance that others have stood where we stand, navigated through the storm, and found peace on the other side. Join us in this journey from wounds to wisdom and discover the power of solidarity in overcoming adversity and embracing healing.*

*With love and gratitude,*
*The Wounds to Wisdom Tribe*

# PRAISES for Wounds to Wisdom: Healing Through Veteran and First Responder Narratives

"*Life is a journey that isn't possible without struggle. What if we could repurpose that struggle into stories to serve others in their darkest moments? That's exactly what Sara Correll and the amazing authors of this book have done on every single page. They've turned wounds into wisdom. I tore through this book like a summer tornado in Kansas, and I know you will too. No matter what challenge in life has scuffed you up, you'll locate yourself in these stories...and more importantly, you'll see a pathway to healing and better days.*"

**~Scott Mann: Former Green Beret,
Founder of Task Force Pineapple,
Best-selling author of Operation Pineapple Epress**

"*Bravery and courage are not the same thing. Bravery leads some people to run into a firefight or a burning building, take a call from someone on the worst day of their life, or endure the long wait while their loved one may be in harm's way on a daily basis. Courage comes from the word coeur in French, which means heart. To be courageous is to reveal what is in your heart. Courage requires a type of moral fortitude that shows up in a willingness to take emotional risks and be vulnerable with others. "Wounds to Wisdom" highlights the stories of 29 protectors and defenders who are both brave, and courageous. Sharing their stories is an extension of their mission to serve — they expose their struggles and lead with hope, so that others can heal.*"

**~Shauna 'Doc' Springer, Ph.D., author of Beyond the Military,
WARRIOR: How to Support Those Who Protect Us and RELENT-
LESS COURAGE: Winning the Battle Against Frontline Trauma**

*"This book will absolutely change your life. These are the most real, authentically raw, vulnerable, and powerful stories shared by The Power of Our Story Tribe. Through the telling of their experiences, this will prove the hardships and struggles you have gone through, make you all that more valuable. Think (Kintsugi Bowl Art)! Trauma is the real cost of the professions we have chosen. The cost doesn't have to take over your life. Together we can take back control and guide the path we take, rather than letting the path guide our journey. This book will help create a path of healing through the darkness. As Jocko Willink says: "Simple Not Easy"."*

**~Sergeant Chris Gregorio - Seattle Police Department
U.S Army Retired MWD Handler**

*"Wounds to Wisdom: Healing Through Veteran and First Responder Narratives" is a transformative masterpiece. As a former Naval Special Warfare Operator, veteran & first responder mental health advocate, I found this book profoundly impactful. It masterfully captures the raw, authentic experiences of those who have served on the front lines. Each narrative is a testament to resilience and the incredible journey from trauma to triumph. This book is not just a collection of stories; it's a beacon of hope, offering invaluable insights into healing and growth. It is a must-read for anyone committed to supporting our brave heroes in their journey to wellness."*

**~Michael Higgs | Navy SEAL (Ret)**

*"These are raw first-hand accounts from those who have been through trauma, who support them, and who are left behind to pick up the pieces. Their vulnerability shows light for those thinking they may be alone. As you read their stories, you'll get a snapshot of their inspiring journeys and realize wounds don't define us. There is hope with wisdom."*

**~Herb Thompson, retired Green Beret,
and author of "The Transition Mission"**

*"Everyone experiences trauma in various forms and degrees—it's an inevitable part of life. This book presents gritty, honest, and powerful stories of people who have walked through the fire, reached the brink, and emerged determined to live fully and support others on their journeys. Facing life's trials alone is not how we're meant to live; life is meant to be shared. From the beginning, as God declared in Genesis 2:18, "It's not good for man to be alone." Through relationships and connection, God transforms what was meant for harm into good. These stories will inspire you to share your own and live the life God uniquely created for you, despite your challenges and trauma."*

**~Rick Wolf, LtCol USMC Retired,
Founder & President, Soul Survivor Outdoor**

*"This is an inspirational book that gives hope. I produced two documentary films featuring interviews with veterans and first responders that were battling post-traumatic stress, but then they found something that changed everything, and allowed them to live a life worth living. There is hope, and what excites me about this book is that each of the personal stories featured are written by people that had difficult struggles in their lives, and now they're sharing how they overcame them. The book is filled with honest and vulnerable stories that prove that you are not alone, and that you can make it through as well."*

**~Michael Gier, Award-Winning Filmmaker**

*"In a world where stories hold immense power, the act of sharing them becomes not just important, but critical. It is through storytelling that healing takes root, nurturing not only the storyteller but all who lend their ears and hearts to listen. The imperative for our war fighters to share their experiences cannot be overstated; it is a vital step towards their healing and our understanding. As citizens of this nation, it is our profound duty to listen, to bear witness to their narratives. Let us embrace this therapeutic exchange of stories with open minds and compassionate hearts, fostering a community bound by empathy and understanding."*

**~Jen Satterly, Author of Arsenal of Hope,
CEO/Founder of All Secure Foundation**

# CONTENTS

Praise for Wounds to Wisdom ............................... vi
Suffering in Silence ...................................... xiii

1. Born to Survive; Rebuilt to Thrive ...................... 1
   *By Deny Caballero, Chief Warrant Officer 2, SF (Ret.)*

2. The Last Breath ........................................ 9
   *By Barry Zworestine, Psychologist, Combat Veteran*

3. The Long Road Home: Finding Purpose in the
   Wreckage ............................................. 17
   *By Jeremy Gronau, Former US Army Apache Helicopter Pilot*

4. Dancing Around the Fire ............................... 26
   *By Steve Giblin, Navy SEAL Master Chief (Ret.)*

5. Coming Home .......................................... 35
   *By Shad Meshad, US Army Capt., Medical Service Corps*

6. The Journey Back to True Empowerment ................. 45
   *By Michelle Franklin, 911 Dispatcher Supervisor (Ret.)*

7. The Day Curiosity Saved My Life ....................... 53
   *By Michael Halterman, Marine Raider (Ret.)*

8. That Others May Live .................................. 59
   *By Glenn Ignazio, Combat Rescue and Special Operations Pilot,
   Major USAF (Ret.)*

9. Two Valleys and a Summit—How Painful
   Journeys Can Forge Beautiful Answers ................... 68
   *By Zeke Vanderpool, U.S. Army Combat Veteran, Federal Agent
   and Mary Millsaps, Creator and Co-Founder of Operation Angel*

10. Choices . . . . . . . . . . . . . . . . . . . . . . . . . . . . . . . . . . . . . . . 80
   *By Justin Wood, Firefighter Paramedic*

11. From Darkness, a Calling . . . . . . . . . . . . . . . . . . . . . . . . . 88
   *By Todd Stewart, Firefighter (Ret.), Chaplain*

12. Choosing Love Over Fear . . . . . . . . . . . . . . . . . . . . . . . . . 97
   *By Holly Higgins, Gold Star Mom of SrA Daniel J Johnson*

13. Carrying His Legacy: A Sister's Journey Through
   Loss and Healing . . . . . . . . . . . . . . . . . . . . . . . . . . . . . . . 106
   *By Melissa Hanks Ketchel, Gold Star Sister of
   LCPL Michael W. Hanks, Veteran Advocate*

14. Our Second Chances . . . . . . . . . . . . . . . . . . . . . . . . . . . . . 114
   *By Scott Duncan, LtCol USMC (Ret.)*

15. Faith, Forgiveness, and Letting Go . . . . . . . . . . . . . . . . . 122
   *By Lona Spisso, Combat Veteran*

16. Silent Battle Cry . . . . . . . . . . . . . . . . . . . . . . . . . . . . . . . . 131
   *By Lakeydra Houston, Master Sargeant (Ret.) US Air Force*

17. Conduct Unbecoming . . . . . . . . . . . . . . . . . . . . . . . . . . . . 140
   *By Robert Ledogar, US Navy, US Marshals Service & Veteran
   Affairs Healthcare (Ret.)*

18. Addiction: The Antithetical Gift . . . . . . . . . . . . . . . . . . . 148
   *By Michael Peyton, Navy SEAL (Ret.)*

19. A Rookie Cop's Longest Ride . . . . . . . . . . . . . . . . . . . . . . 157
   *By Rich Oakley, DEA Senior Special Agent (Ret.)*

20. The Wisdom of Forgiveness . . . . . . . . . . . . . . . . . . . . . . . 166
   *By Chad Bruckner, Police Officer and Army Veteran*

21. Unpacking My Emotional Rucksack ........................ 174
    *By Daniel Torrez, Combat Veteran, Advocate, Servant Leader*

22. The Last to Abandon ............................... 183
    *By Christopher Hoyer, Police Officer (Ret.), Advocate*

23. When the Mask Cracked, Everything Changed ............. 191
    *By Janet Wiszowaty, Emergency Dispatcher (Ret.), Royal*
    *Canadian Mounted Police*

24. The Fire Service: The Test of One Man's Mettle .......... 199
    *By Jim Lydon, Fire Chief (Ret.)*

25. Earn Your Badge Every Day .......................... 207
    *By David Berez Police Officer (Ret.)*

26. Grit, Gratitude, and Grace ........................... 216
    *By Michael DeSelm, USN Veteran, Dive Med Tech,*
    *Veteran Advocate*

27. Embracing Crisis: A Journey of Growth, Resilience,
    and Faith ......................................... 225
    *By Michael Pellegrino, Detective (Ret.)*

28. Ya Gotta OWN Your Condition! ........................ 234
    *By Gregg F. Martin, Major General, US Army (Ret.)*


Acknowledgements ......................................... 244
About The Editor ......................................... 246
About the Author ......................................... 251

# SUFFERING IN SILENCE

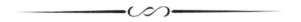

*An Introduction*

In 2003, I was organizing my office. With one baby down for a nap and our other two boys at school, the telephone rang. It was my mother. She said straight away, "Sara, I have bad news; you need to sit down." She then proceeded to share that my dad had died by suicide.

*What?!*

I heard the words, but I couldn't wrap my mind around what they meant. The world started moving in slow motion, as I tried to comprehend what I just heard. I was devastated. My mind, soul, and spirit were crushed. In the blink of an eye, I was altered forever and forced to start a journey of learning how to function in my new world.

*My dad!? Suicide!?*

Who is ever prepared for this? And what do you do when your world changes in one second, and the expectations of life keep moving forward, faster than ever? I was bombarded by the what ifs and whys. What should I (or could I) have done? And how could I handle the shame of being unable to remember simple things in my daily schedule?

*Was I losing it?*

Later that year, my husband and I had a fourth son. What a joy he was to our family! He never stopped smiling. He was born with a little birthmark on his head in the shape of a cross; it served as a reminder to me that there is always hope. I latched onto my faith in God, and it anchored me in love, hope and healing.

Bad times don't last forever, but the journey through can be long and lonely. Daily, I was fighting to muster the energy to act "normal." It was compounded with the little sleep I got after having a new baby and three other little boys to look after. I did my best, as I wanted my kids to love their childhood. We had a lot of fun, but I was still suffering inside. I wasn't free.

When the kids got older, I had a burning passion to help those who were suffering in silence to not feel so alone as they navigated their lonely journey to healing. I didn't know what that looked like or what population I could best serve. I asked myself; what if I could help alleviate some of the pain and shame from those suffering souls trying to put on a brave smile every day? So much energy is needed to smile when you just feel like crying. It is exhausting to keep up a brave face, on top of everything else.

I initially started a book club on healing, gathering women who also needed a safe place to share their stories and struggles. I looked forward to it so much every week; it was the only place outside of my family and close friends that I could let down my guard. I felt safe and cared for, and the other women did, too. I witnessed the power of connection and healing in those gatherings. Years later, I opened our home to feed our sons' friends and teammates during sports seasons. I would make a big pot of chicken tortilla soup every week, providing them a safe place to gather. An assistant football coach would come over and go deep, inviting the boys to share how their lives were going and making sure to check in with everyone. The tears, the laughter, and the camaraderie were powerful! This became a tradition with three out of four of our sons; I fed kids every week for eleven years.

These experiences (and a big pot of chicken tortilla soup) taught me so much about the importance of fellowship, having a place of safety to share our life and stories, and the healing power of showing up authentically in a community that cares and is rooting for you—always! Storytelling, in particular, has a way of healing both the teller and the listener. In releasing and sharing our stories with others, as well as hearing others articulate their own journey of trauma and healing, we gain understanding and insight. That is what grew inside me; the idea that there is powerful healing that happens in community that allows for bonding through sharing stories.

When the boys were almost grown, I went back to school to become a counselor. One day I found myself sitting next to a Veteran in class. Curious, I asked if he would share his story with me. Hearing his story bubbled up a deep compassion and understanding for him and connection with my own story of suffering. It opened my eyes and my heart, and it fueled my passion to support those who signed on that line and swore an oath to protect us, even on their worst day. From that point on, I wanted to be there for our Protectors.

When I read the statistics of suicide for our Veterans, First Responders, and all our Protectors, I was deeply moved and concerned, wanting to understand more. I felt so connected to those who had sacrificed and were suffering in silence. So many are dealing with physical, spiritual, and moral injury. And those who are no longer active duty are missing their tribe, their way of life, their mission, and purpose. I wanted to do something about it. I wanted to protect our Protectors. I had so many questions, like where is the "reboot" camp for those leaving the military, to help reintegrate back into society when they entered at such a young age? Why are those who have sacrificed so much to protect us dying by suicide? Why are those who protected us suffering so silently? And why are civilians like me so disconnected from the cost of war? Somehow, through my own life experience, our Protectors and their challenges made sense to me.

It all began when one Veteran started coming over to my house to share his story. I would invite people in my community over to listen and hear him speak. Thereby, coming closer to the cost of war, as well as welcoming him into civilian life. I wanted to create a safe place for those who have served and are suffering in silence. I wanted to create a platform where our Protectors could connect, be seen and heard in a judgment-free zone, where others were on the same journey.

Taking one brave step forward starts the healing process. Releasing our stories connects us and, again, it helps us gain insight into our own stories. Sharing our stories is so important when we've experienced trauma or profound grief, such as losing our tribe, losing our "normal," seeing or experiencing something that causes moral injury.

I got on LinkedIn the week the world shut down in March of 2020. I asked if there were any Veterans who wanted to have a conversation. From that point, there was an explosion of connection and born from it a network of Protectors who are there for each other. We have weekly virtual Coffee and Conversation groups called The Power Of Our Story. Together, everyone builds the tribe of healing. I found the work to be a good fit and loved the resilience I saw while healing.

Today, my husband (of 34 years) and I are now grandparents. Our family is close, and we are living our best life. I'm so grateful! It is amazing how the worst thing that can happen in life can be the very thing that empowers us to care so deeply for others. The suffering can create a deep desire for a new mission of service. Life is messy, and it can be unbelievably hard, but never, never, never give up!

It has been an honor and a pleasure to see our Protectors regain their confidence and remember who they are. The badge and uniform did not make them; they made the badge and uniform. They take those strengths to the next season of Purpose and Mission.

*Wounds to Wisdom: Healing Through Veteran and First Responder Narratives* evolved from so many Protectors willing to step up and share their stories, connect, and "be there" for one another on The Power Of Our Story, and through connections made on LinkedIn. I am inspired and grateful for my Protector brothers and sisters. I love you, and I appreciate you. There are SO MANY who helped build this tribe; I can't even begin to thank everyone individually.

The Power Of Our Story is all about protecting and connecting our Protectors, those who have been well trained in every way, with the exception of what to do with trauma and what to expect when transitioning/retiring. So many leave themselves behind after transitioning, perhaps isolating, not allowing their body, mind, soul, and spirit to heal when all the events of active duty start bubbling up. The Power Of Our Story is a place where vetted resources and alternative modalities are discussed. It is a place where the words "me too" forge family and friendship from faraway places.

And to the one holding this book, I know it may not feel like it at times, but you are not alone. Really. The best thing you can do for yourself is take one small, courageous step forward every day. Whatever that looks like for you. I hope as you read these authors' stories, you connect to their pain, their trauma, their grief, and their betrayal. I hope you glean from how they faced their challenges, mustered the courage to move forward, and started sharing their stories with others.

I encourage you to consider writing down your own thoughts after each story. What came up for you after hearing from each author? Can you relate? What emotions are coming up for you overall? Consider writing it all down. Then, think about how these authors reframed their stories so the healing process could begin and ignite resiliency. Moreover, reach out to these authors and their non-profits if you need support or want to connect. Take that brave step. The resources and vetted healing modalities are here for you in the pages of this book.

You're worth it. Your family is worth it. Please don't suffer in silence; there is hope.

∾

*We love you.*
*We see you.*
*We believe in you.*
*We pray you find healing in these lived stories.*

∾

*With love and respect,*
*Sara Correll*

# CHAPTER 1
# BORN TO SURVIVE; REBUILT TO THRIVE

*By*

*Deny Caballero*

Green Berets are the masters of tackling the unconventional, the complex, and what others view as the impossible. From the beginning of our training, we are taught to focus only on accomplishing the mission. As a Green Beret, this singular focus mindset ruled over my life. Nothing else mattered, not my health, family, or personal relationships. Only the mission. Yet, avoidance had always been part of my life. I grew up as an extremely abused child. I endured years of sexual, physical, and mental abuse at the hands of my biological mother and stepfather. The first time I thought I was going to die wasn't in combat, it was as a six-year-old child, as my stepfather wrapped his hands around my neck and slowly choked me to the point that I passed out. I lived in a constant state of "fight, flight, or freeze." Yet from May 1991 until June 2002, my life was a constant whirlwind of abuse and near-death encounters at the hands of a sick and sadistic child predator.

Humans don't break like they do in war movies. It took years to dismantle my mental well-being. I had avoided, disassociated, and neglected every aspect of my trauma, both civilian and combat. By 2019, I had already deployed twice to Iraq during "the Surge" and once to Afghanistan. I had lost friends, experienced combat as a Green Beret, and endured multiple injuries during training and on deployments—the worst being multiple concussions due to Airborne operations, blast wave exposure, and a fused neck. Concussions are nonpenetrative or penetrative traumatic brain injuries, yet no one takes them seriously, unless you have brain matter leaking out or you can't move. But jumping isn't the only culprit; shooting heavy weapons, mortars, .50 cal sniper rifles and, yes, even the "Carl G", officially known as SRAAW (M), (Short-Range Anti-Armour Weapon-Medium), if shot enough can scramble your brain. I didn't know that, and I definitely didn't notice the impact until everything else started coming undone.

In 2020, after my last combat trip to Afghanistan, I fell apart —rapidly. I was breaking down physically, emotionally, spiritually, and mentally. The catalyst for this rapid breakdown was my chronic pain and my declining cognitive function. I couldn't walk, stand, or move without excruciating pain in both of my feet. Deep searing pain shot through my feet, legs, and lower back. I dealt with this pain all throughout the deployment, and in order to function, I relied on multiple shots of Toradol on a daily basis. Back at home though, I wasn't able to receive anything for the pain. The pain was unimaginable, but the lack of cognitive function was worse.

Mission requirements don't let up in Special Forces. Shortly after returning home, I was already planning our next trip. Pre-deployment training, budgets, ammunition allocations, pre-deployment surveys, projected manning, and trying to navigate my own life became an impossible task. I started having issues concentrating, staring at emails for hours not knowing what I was reading. My memory and retention were no longer reliable. I would get lost going home or drive for hours not knowing where I was going. Suddenly, my own memory couldn't be trusted. I would blame my wife for moving my items around, only to find them hours later in random parts of the house. At work, I was functioning at my maximum capacity but failing miserably to uphold the standards of the Regiment. I was killing myself trying to do what used to be so easy. My overall health continued to decline. At times, my left eye would not focus. I was experiencing severe panic attacks. I couldn't sleep, and I was suffering from debilitating migraines.

It had been a year since I got back from that last trip, and my life had become a complete act of desperation. It had been over a year, and I was no closer to getting better. In my desperation, I agreed to have surgeries on both of my feet. After months of rehabilitation and treatment, I was still in constant pain. I had started seeing one of the behavioral health counselors at my unit, yet I never fully divulged any of my trauma, only half-truths. Eventually, I was referred to a neuropsychologist to identify what was going on with me cognitively. After numerous tests, the doctor identified that I was dealing with a multitude of issues, resulting from multiple nonpenetrative, traumatic brain injuries. The doctor reassured me that I would be okay and that I would adapt. Yet it was very clear that there was no going back to the person I once was. I didn't want to adapt. I didn't want a new life, and I didn't want to give up control.

After that doctor's visit, I was a broken man, clinging to an identity that was becoming too heavy to uphold. I would still sit with my counselor, Michelle, at P3 (the mental health clinic), but nothing changed. I still danced around the truth and what I was dealing with. I couldn't keep up with the demands at work. Physically, I couldn't do what a Green Beret is supposed to do, and at home, I was failing as a husband. I was angry, resentful, filled with shame and guilt that I was not living up to the standards of a Special Forces soldier. I didn't want a new life. I wanted to go out as a proud and strong Green Beret.

I had no intention of telling Michelle anything, but somehow during one of our talks, I found myself having my first real moment of vulnerability. I admitted to something I never thought I would. For months, I'd been waiting for my wife to deploy. I planned to end my life while she was away. Michelle saved my life that day. She helped me see a way through what I was feeling, and then she helped get me into a mental health treatment center. That one, brief moment of vulnerability changed my life forever. This was the turning point for me.

The tools that helped me on my journey were not easy to identify at first. After much debate and analysis, I settled on these four key components: *vulnerability*, *self-advocacy*, *courage*, and *self-compassion*. These four factors changed me deeply, and it is my belief that they can do the same for you.

**Vulnerability** is the first attribute that allowed me to actually get help. I didn't want to be seen as broken. To me, the idea of being vulnerable meant exposing myself to more trauma, to more pain, and worst of all … judgement. When I actually told Michelle my full truth and the extent of my suffering in my first true moment of vulnerability, I wasn't ridiculed, laughed at or made to feel less than. Instead, I was given resources that helped me in my time of need. It was that first bold step toward vulnerability that helped save my life and set me on a course toward healing.

**Self-advocacy** is something most of us are very bad at doing. From the moment we arrive at basic training, we are taught to keep our mouths shut and to only speak when spoken to. In the world of Special Operations, we take this to the extreme. As I started healing, I realized if I wanted to continue getting access to care, I had to be the one to ask for treatment, resources, and better care. Many of us are looking for others to do the asking, whether it's a spouse or patient advocate. Self-advocacy was being willing to fight for myself. I didn't need someone else to rescue me; I simply needed to do the work.

*Courage* is a value that every service member knows and has demonstrated during their time in service. Yet the version of courage that helped me on my journey is not the same. The courage I'm talking about is the courage to go into the unknown in healing and recovery. We think that courage is only found in faraway lands in the middle of war zones, but that's not true. On my mental health journey, I have had to lean into the unknown, the uncomfortable, and painful in order to stay on my course. Courage is being willing to face the unknown and doing what's necessary to heal.

Lastly, the single greatest component to this mission is **self-compassion**. Many will start the healing process with the idea that they are doing it for someone else, but the truth is the healing has to be done for you. Before we can love and care for others, we must care for and love ourselves. Mental health is a long and ever-winding journey. If you're just starting yours, I urge you to try some of the tools I used. Above all, learn to fall in love with the process of improvement. Fall in love with doing the work.

# MEET DENY CABALLERO

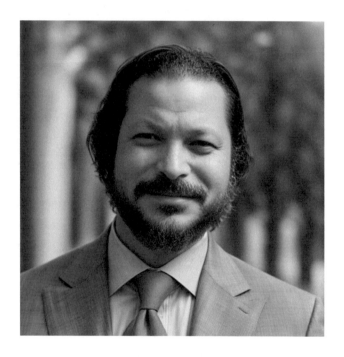

CW2(ret.) Deny Caballero was born in Panama, Central America and is a proud, first-generation American. As a child, Deny suffered and endured significant trauma at the hands of his parents, yet even at a young age, he knew he was meant for more.

Deny served in the 82$^{nd}$ Airborne Division. After two year-long deployments, he attended the Special Forces Assessment and Selection course, where he successfully completed SFAS and graduated the Qualification course in May of 2012 as a Special Forces Weapons Sergeant.

As a Green Beret, Deny served with great distinction, setting himself apart from his peers through his work ethic, tenacious spirit, and "Never Quit!" outlook. In 2017, he volunteered once again; this time, it was to become a Special Forces Warrant Officer.

Serving as a Special Forces Chief Warrant Officer was the highlight of his career, and he exemplified what it meant to be a "Chief." As a Combat leader, Deny never missed a mission and always took the point man position, ensuring that he always led from the front. Throughout his career, he endured numerous injuries and health issues, which led to a medical retirement.

Deny uses the lessons and skills that he learned while serving as a Green Beret to help inspire others to achieve greatness and to help create positive change wherever he is called to serve. As a leader in the Veteran community, Deny hopes to inspire others to reach for the impossible and live to succeed again.

∾

### Connect with Deny
#### Chief Warrant Officer 2. SF (Ret.)

*Email: deny.caballero@securityhalt.com*
*LinkedIn: Deny Caballero*
*Website: www.securityhalt.com*
*Listen in to: Security Halt! Podcast*

∾

# Your Turn

What came up for you in this story?

_____

_____

_____

_____

_____

_____

_____

_____

_____

_____

_____

_____

_____

_____

_____

_____

_____

_____

_____

_____

_____

_____

_____

_____

_____

# CHAPTER 2
## THE LAST BREATH

———— ∽ ————

*By*
*Barry Zworestine*

He lay still on the table. I could barely hear his breath. It was 0200 (2:00 a.m.) in 1976 while on high density force operations in a four man stick in the Rhodesian Bush War. After I had put out the flames, his body was blackened and burnt following the ambush that we removed him from. I was unable to get a tube down his throat. I stood there, helpless, in the stillness of the night in our bush camp. There was nothing I could do to save him. He suddenly took one long, deep breath in, filling his lungs. Then slowly the breath, his last raspy breath, released itself from his body. It seemed to go on forever as it slowly drifted away over the tops of the trees, leaving his body blackened, rigid, and still on the table.

Forty-seven years later, I still hear that last breath. It has never left me. It has lived within me, like a memory of a distant time, in a war that claimed so many lives. It speaks to me of that place between life and death. My war did not end as I struggled through five emigrations and losses that impacted me deeply, affecting my family, my relationships, and others who died under my hands as I tried to save them.

It took a large portion of my life to realize that underlying all my journeys and challenges was a deep pool of unresolved grief, a numbing sadness that felt like a thick skin growing around my heart, damping down my capacity to feel joy. Although I functioned well as a teacher and later as a psychologist, I felt that I had lost pieces of myself, bit by bit, over the years. Each unresolved loss and memory seemed to take more from me. Grief was (and still is) not something I easily embrace. It can feel too overwhelming.

So, I began to run. First, short runs and half-marathons then marathons and ultramarathons. I would run on trails where I found peace in my body as it moved in nature, the ground beneath my feet, surrounded by trees and the stillness of my breath. I found my peace running in extreme heat, pushing hard to my extremes to the place where life could meet death. It never stopped. To stop would be to feel. So, at sixty-seven, I was pushing my heart to two-hundred beats a minute, tasting the edge of heat stroke.

I have, over time, understood the potentially deadly seduction of chasing the edge. I realized I could never outrun my loss and grief. Those feelings lay quiet, unchanged, and dormant deep within myself, patiently waiting for life and circumstances to call me back to my heart. Something had to change for me to really heal. That something took two forms—the first was bursting a disc two years after my ultramarathon which severed my ability to chase the miles. The second was in 2020 when I blew my meniscus and could no longer run.

In my life journey, chasing my last breath, I have always been disciplined maintaining excellent nutrition, and forty-seven years of meditation. Over the past few years, I have understood the importance of maintaining a certain level of comfort within the discomfort. It helps keep my edge sharp and reminds me that I have not yet lost my fire and passion for living with meaning and purpose. I have maintained three years of cold-water showers and a daily discipline of exercise. But I have also become more willing to feel the edges of my grief. At seventy, I am still a work in progress.

There have been numerous moments over the years that have opened the doors to my grief and loss. At times, this has interwoven with pain and anger. I am aware of a constant level of vigilance and watchfulness. It's like an internal app, quietly burning away inside me and absorbing energy and vitality. It comes and goes, depending on what is happening in my life. But I no longer see this as a destructive force. What I have discovered, as I navigate through my loss and grief, is that there is a gift within this place. I began to hold its presence in my life. My grief and memories of loss and death have awakened in me a mission for service and a compassion and gratitude for what I have in my life.

My journey into service began in 2002 when I started sitting with Veterans and those currently serving. I have seen the immense healing power of service and where present, faith. Now, I am better at making choices that do not place me at risk and that allow me to grow and heal. I will always be grateful to the "last breath" of those I have been privileged to sit with. These breaths whisper to me and guide me forward with gratitude, an open heart and love for the Veterans who are my brothers. As much as I have impacted their lives, they have transformed mine. I am a better man, person, husband, and friend as a result of the extraordinary individuals who traveled and battled through their wars. My challenges still remain, but they are fertile, not barren. I no longer run away from my heart but choose to run into it.

At seventy, I am increasingly aware of my relationship with time. I am grateful for more of the precious moments in my life. I feel the changes in my body and experience limitation, but I am also learning to see the time I have left as an opportunity to leave gifts behind once I, too, have breathed my last breath. The clock is ticking, but each second offers powerful moments, invitations, and opportunities to find gratitude and love and heal pain and grief and grasp the courage, will, and determination to do what needs to be done rather than shrink away from and still my heart.

Change, transformation, and healing have not come easily for me, but I have been willing to hunt for, fight for, and sweat for it. I have learned to listen to the whispers of that which lies in the shadows of my heart and that will often touch me in the early hours of the morning. I know now that this cannot be forgotten, silenced, or locked away. At times, I am aware that my journey can be painful and that I need to draw on my courage, faith, and commitment. I know that it is better to feel than to numb out or push down. I am aware that I can no longer run from change. I am more willing to creak, groan, and stretch into the process. I see how letting go of my wellbeing is also letting go of life. I see the need to greet the moments in my life, take each breath as a gift that deserves gratitude and an investment of time and presence.

And being married to an extraordinary woman for the past ten years, I have experienced life not just as a battle ground of extreme adventure, change, and challenge but as a gentle process of love and feeling safe in the presence of another and allowing my heart to soften and open. I sense that this will continue to be a journey of healing until I breathe my last breath.

∾

To pull this all together I'd like to share what I have learned:

1. As much as I have made others my mission, it is as important to make myself my own personal mission.
2. As much as I would never leave someone behind, I have learned the importance of not leaving myself behind.
3. I will maintain a daily discipline of care no matter how small, whether it be making my bed, eating well, or taking a cold shower.
4. Becoming comfortable with discomfort has allowed me to face what I often chose to ignore or run away from. Building on these moments has taught me confidence, trust in myself, and resilience.
5. I draw on the comfort of my tribe and reach out when I am struggling.
6. At times when my life may feel overwhelming, I can always sit, take a breath then get up, dust myself off, and keep moving forward—one small step at a time.
7. I am worth the effort to recover the positive qualities of who I was and who I am still.
8. I know that my grief will not kill me and that in my grief lies my healing.
9. It is never too late to change, nor am I too old to give up on life.
10. Every breath is an opportunity for service and compassion to self and others.

# MEET BARRY ZWORESTINE

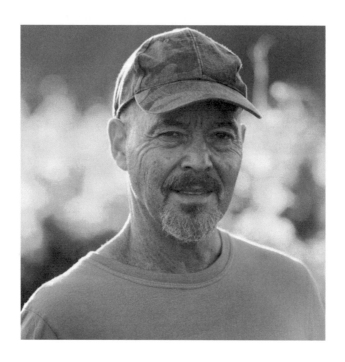

*"No Veteran should ever have to come home to die."*

Barry Zworestine, author of *Which Way Is Your Warrior Facing—An operational manual for current serving and Veterans transitioning into civilian life*, fought as a combat medic in a four-man stick in the Rhodesian Bush War from 1976 to 1977. Since 2002, he has worked as a psychologist with Veterans and those currently serving in Australia. Barry was a marathon and ultramarathon runner who is passionate about music. He plays the African drum, American Indian flute, and the Australian didgeridoo. He is married to an extraordinary woman.

~

### Connect with Barry
**Psychologist, Combat Veteran,**

**Author of Which Way is Your Warrior Facing?: An operational manual for current serving and Veterans transitioning into civilian life**

*Email: navigateforveterans@gmail.com*
*LinkedIn: Barry Zworestine*

~

# Your Turn

What came up for you in this story?

_____

_____

_____

_____

_____

_____

_____

_____

_____

_____

_____

_____

_____

_____

_____

_____

_____

_____

_____

_____

_____

_____

_____

_____

_____

_____

# CHAPTER 3
# THE LONG ROAD HOME: FINDING PURPOSE IN THE WRECKAGE,

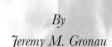

*By*

*Jeremy M. Gronau*

In the tapestry of life, we are often marked by moments of overwhelming adversity, yet it is in the aftermath of such trials that our true strength emerges. Before I drew my first breath, the battle was already underway. My entrance into the world was shadowed by sacrifice; my mother's choice to delay cancer treatment to give me life ultimately cost her own. Growing up with the knowledge that my birth was intertwined with my mother's death burdened my young heart with a profound sense of loss and a quest for understanding. This early confrontation with life's fragility planted seeds of doubt about God's goodness amidst suffering. Yet, it also set the stage for a journey through the darkness towards an unforeseen light, a testament to the enduring power of faith, hope, and the strength of the human soul.

An undercurrent of grief and unanswered questions marked my childhood. The loss of my mother before I could even know her left a void filled with whys and what-ifs. This internal struggle was a constant companion as I navigated life that seemed to compound over time. The decision to join the Army emerged not just as a path to honor the legacy of sacrifice my mother left behind, but as a quest for identity and purpose. My acceptance into flight school marked the beginning of a new chapter. There, amid the rigors of military training, I met my wife, Amanda. Our bond, forged in the demanding test of military life, became my anchor. Upon completing flight school, the call to serve in Afghanistan arrived, a call I answered. I was thrust into the realities of heavy combat, where the stakes of life and death colored every moment. This environment, while deepening my sense of purpose, also magnified the stress and weight of the responsibilities resting on my shoulders.

After my deployment, serving as an Apache helicopter pilot with Charlie Troop, 3-17 Cavalry in the 3rd Infantry Division, I yearned for a peaceful homecoming. Yet, a cascade of personal chaos swiftly overshadowed my anticipated peace. My health deteriorated, affecting me physically, mentally, and spiritually. I endured debilitating pain from arthritis in my knees and shoulders, compounded by herniated discs in my neck and back that compressed my spinal cord. The invisible wounds of PTSD manifested as severe insomnia and a deepening depression. A profound crisis of faith intensified my distress. These challenges set a backdrop of turmoil, where anger and hopelessness became my constant companions. My pursuit of healing led me down countless avenues, from self-help gurus to medical experts, yet peace continued to elude me. In my quest for healing, a Bible study group became my refuge, guiding me to a path I had never considered.

On December 23, 2019, my life's trajectory veered off course in an instant, transforming a family ski trip into a dire emergency when our car hydroplaned and collided with a tree at a terrifying speed. The impact was catastrophic, plunging me into unconsciousness, leaving my wife and two children in peril, and changing our lives forever. We were all trapped inside our smoking vehicle, a living nightmare unfolding around us. Amanda was engulfed in a haze of pain and confusion, covered in broken glass. Coming to amidst the wreckage, her first heart-wrenching thought as she looked at me crushed in the driver seat was that I had perished. Confronted with her own severe injuries —both hands and wrists shattered, leaving her powerless to move or aid our children—she was in intense despair.

Quick-thinking, good Samaritans, witnessing the aftermath, sprang into action, shattering the back window to free my children from the smoldering vehicle. With the arrival of the paramedics, they discovered me in the throes of a convulsive seizure. My legs were crushed beneath the dashboard and crumpled metal of the vehicle, a litany of fractures and injuries were etched across my upper body. It took First Responders thirty minutes to extract me from the twisted embrace of the car using the jaws of life. This accident, horrific in every sense, became the crucible for an unforeseen transformation.

Days later, following several surgeries, I found myself awaiting a transfer to Grady Memorial Hospital. There, the director of Orthopedic Trauma planned to undertake the delicate task of reconstructing my right leg. On New Year's Eve, in the solitude of my hospital room, I gazed out at the Appalachian Mountains. The realization dawned on me that my physical injuries and the heavy burden of guilt for endangering my family due to my reckless driving in the rain were formidable mountains I had yet to climb. Confronted with overwhelming hopelessness and shame, I sought the Lord's guidance and strength, pleading for His assistance in navigating the daunting path ahead. In this moment of isolation, I turned to Him in prayer.

After my transfer to Grady, Dr. Schenker briefed me on the high risks of my upcoming surgery to repair my severely fractured tibia, describing it as one of the worst cases she'd encountered. The morning of my surgery, I wrestled with my nerves, thinking it might be my final moments. I decided to take one last picture of myself before being put under. As I was wheeled into the brightly lit operating room, filled with a team of medical professionals, the opening notes of a familiar song filled the space. As "Spirit in the Sky" began playing from a speaker on the wall, the timing of the song choice and the irony of its lyrics at that moment did not escape me. It was as if God had created this moment for my benefit alone. A nurse smiled at me and said, "Perfect song for an Apache pilot."

In that vulnerable state, surrounded by medical equipment and the muted conversations of the surgical team, I turned inward, reaching out to God in a way I hadn't done before. I acknowledged the years I had spent distancing myself from His guidance, the silent rebellion of a heart that chose to wander.

With the melody echoing softly in the background, I surrendered fully to the divine, relinquishing control of my life and the outcome of the surgery. My prayer was simple yet profound: if I woke up from this ordeal, it would be with a heart renewed in faith, with Jesus firmly at its center. It was a request for a second chance, not just at life but at a life lived purposefully and by His will. I experienced a profound sense of peace and calm. At that moment, I felt the presence of something divine, a comforting assurance whispering through the depths of my soul: "Everything is exactly as it should be."

Waking up in the ICU after an eight-hour surgery, I faced the harsh reality of my state. Despite significant blood loss and the searing pain that gripped me, the sight of both my feet at the end of my bed brought a profound sense of relief and gratitude. Reflecting on the pre-surgery events, I remembered the photo I had taken just before being wheeled into the operating room. Looking at the picture, I noticed a big digital clock over my right shoulder. The clock read 7:07. This sparked a compelling thought, urging me to consult The Book of Matthew. With anticipation, I opened the Bible app on my phone. As I read chapter seven, verse seven, tears streamed down my face, overwhelmed by the profound message.

"Ask and it will be given to you; seek and you will find; knock and the door will be opened to you. For everyone who asks receives; the one who seeks finds; and to the one who knocks, the door will be opened. Which of you, if your son asks for bread, will give him a stone? Or if he asks for a fish, will give him a snake? If you, then, though you are evil, know how to give good gifts to your children, how much more will your Father in heaven give good gifts to those who ask Him!" *(Matthew 7:7-11)*\*

Emerging from this trial, I was not the same person. My physical recovery, which took years and was marked by a series of grueling surgeries, mirrored my spiritual rebirth. This harrowing experience not only deepened my faith but also granted me a fresh perspective on life, transforming my pain into a wellspring of strength and compassion. This transformation led me to pursue a career in Christian counseling and high-performance coaching, aiming to support Veterans, First Responders, and trauma survivors through their most challenging times, offering a comprehensive approach to personal and professional development. My journey from despair to hope, from soldier to counselor, is a testament to God's providential design for each of our lives, the power of faith, and the resilience of the human spirit.

---

\*   Matthew 7:7-11, New International Version

It is a message of hope for those wrestling with their own adversities, a reminder that even in our darkest hour, we are never alone. My path has led me to a calling where I can be a beacon of light for others, guiding them through their storms toward a horizon filled with light and new beginnings.

"The Lord your God is with you, the Mighty Warrior who saves. He will take great delight in you; in His love, He will no longer rebuke you but will rejoice over you with singing." *(Zephaniah 3:17)* *

---

\* Zephaniah 3:17, New International Version

# MEET JEREMY GRONAU

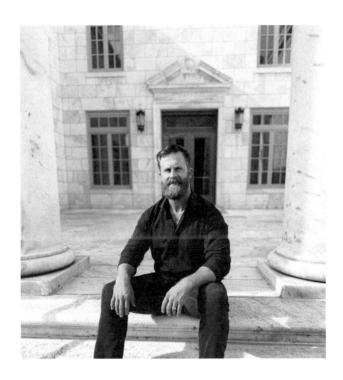

Jeremy Gronau's life is a powerful chronicle of sacrifice, survival, and spiritual awakening. From the adrenaline-charged atmosphere of an Apache Helicopter Attack Squadron navigating aerial combat in Afghanistan to his calling as a devoted Christian counselor, Jeremy harnesses his military experience and spiritual insights to confront the unseen battles of the heart, mind, and spirit. With a radiating empathy that heals the wounded soul, he inspires excellence through strategic coaching and direction. As a seasoned leader with over 15 years of rigorous management and operational expertise, his mission is to accompany people from the depths of pain to the pinnacle of peace, from the echoes of wounds to wisdom and revival. Grounded in the teachings of Jesus Christ and powered by a fortified faith in God, he draws on the "Warrior Spirit" philosophy, igniting hope in those seeking restoration. If you feel moved by Jeremy's story and mission or seek guidance on your path to healing and personal excellence, feel free to reach out to him.

∾

### *Connect with Jeremy*
**Former US Army Apache Helicopter Pilot,**

**Christian Counselor, and High-Performance Coach**

*Email: jeremy@warriorsinchrist.one*
*LinkedIn: Jeremy Gronau*
*Website: www.warriorsinchrist.one*

∾

# Your Turn

What came up for you in this story?

_____
_____
_____
_____
_____
_____
_____
_____
_____
_____
_____
_____
_____
_____
_____
_____
_____
_____
_____
_____
_____
_____

# CHAPTER 4
# DANCING AROUND THE FIRE

*By*
*Steve Giblin*

I joined the Navy in 1981, at the tender age of seventeen. After a deployment and one-year tour on the aircraft carrier USS Ranger, I was granted orders to BUD/S, Basic Underwater Demolition/SEAL Training where I learned the basics of being a Frogman, aka "Navy SEAL." I spent the next twenty-six years in the Teams, bouncing around the globe, conducting special operations, training with foreign partner special operations units, and forward deploying for contingency operations. I operated mini-wet-submersibles from submarines and surface ships, conducted more than 1,200 military parachute drops, and was a member of SEAL Team Six for fourteen years. I was a Command Master Chief (senior enlisted advisor) at two Naval Special Warfare commands, finishing out my career in San Diego, where I started, at BUD/S as a Phase Master Chief and then as the Operations Master Chief before retiring from active duty in 2009.

After retirement, I continued to work for my community, serving as a contractor and then as a government civil service employee for nine years. After thirty-seven years of combined service, my wife and I hung it all up and retired for good. She's also retired active duty (a Navy Chief Petty Officer and civil service employee). We're now living in the Southwest where we plan on calling the desert home.

Blowing things up for a living and sustaining at least three known concussions is the root cause of many problems in my life. Unbeknownst to me and many of my comrades, blast exposure, heavy weapons and the opening shock of a parachute causes brain injury. Microscopic tears that aren't detected in an MRI or CT scan create what I call a "wiring problem in the brain housing unit." The medical profession calls it traumatic brain injury (TBI), damage caused because of a sudden, forceful impact or jolt to the head. The symptoms from this injury range from mild to severe, involving confusion, impaired motor skills, chronic headaches, depression, cognitive and memory issues, and sometimes suicide.

There is also chronic traumatic encephalopathy (CTE), also a result of repetitive blast exposure, often experienced by military personnel. Blast-related CTE shares similarities to traditional CTE, like the kind seen in NFL players, but it's distinguished by the unique impact of shockwaves on the brain. Military Veterans, particularly Special Operations Forces (SOF), whose main job it is to train for combat and forward deploy into combat zones, may be at an increased risk of developing blast related CTE.

Special Operations Forces (SOF) training is mentally, emotionally, and physically demanding. It includes intensive operational training, simulating harsh combat and combat deployment cycles. I spent eleven years out of twenty-eight deployed overseas. My experience wasn't as intense as the younger generations', but the training remains the same, in and out of the schoolhouse (i.e., formal training in basic or advanced skillsets around explosives, parachutes, etc.). The US Navy deploys routinely, not just to go into combat but to provide presence, deterrence, and nation partner building with foreign counterparts. SEAL Teams are no different.

After retiring from active duty, I started noticing problems. My wife will tell you; she saw my struggles years before, shortly after we married. Explosive anger, forgetfulness, and sleeplessness. The problems I noticed were lack of sleep and depression. I associated the latter with the lack of sleep, so I focused on getting a better night's rest.

I tailored my workouts to a more consistent rhythm with breaks for yoga and chilling out. The sleep problems continued. I drank more, wine mostly, but could down plenty of beer. I could kill a bottle of wine, no problem. I'd tell myself, "Self-control, Steven!"

Fortunately (and unfortunately), my work as a civilian with the SEAL Teams lead to more internal conflict—I missed deployments and the close-knit camaraderie. Deployment was what we always trained for—war or not. Not being deployed also disturbed my sleep. Fear of Missing Out (FOMO).

I was having difficulty with my new life as a civilian, managing my worry, ruminating, and handling stressful situations in new ways. I discovered the cultures and demands of civilian life was vastly different from the military. Relaxing at night when it was time to sleep, only caused my brain to wander and worry, keeping me awake. I had also suffered from hyper-vigilance. I was told I was on guard all the time. My memory problems meant missing appointments and meetings. My work faltered, which disturbed me enormously. That wasn't me! I was always "Mr. Johnny on the Spot." Sticky-notes started appearing everywhere, reminding me to do this and that. It was frustrating, infuriating at times. And I felt a lot of shame for that.

Honestly, I didn't experience anything terrible in any of my combat deployments.

I went.

I did.

And I returned.

The training I experienced was always more difficult and intense than just about any deployment I ever made. That was part of my shame as well — *I didn't suffer enough*.

Life outside the military is typically more mundane, lacking the stimulus of life-and-death situations. Critical ingredients to human health and well-being include a sense of purpose, daily structured activities, and a continued sense of earned success and contribution. Work is one of the most important aspects of human life, yet most SOF operators struggle—at least for a while —to develop satisfying post-military career paths. Many operators also struggle with the loss of purpose, loss of "tribe," and reintegration into their own homes, families, and communities.

There's the fear of developing "invisible wounds." As the number of operators and operations increases, people I know who have committed suicide or self-destructed in other ways (i.e., substance abuse, risky behaviors), and as the evidence grows regarding the significant toll taken by traumatic brain injury (TBI), I quietly wonder if I will be next.

There's a pervasive awareness within the SOF community that the "invisible wounds" of war, including chronic traumatic encephalopathy (CTE), may claim them, too. Part of my dread, the rumination of who I will hear about next. Or will it be me who is next?

I won't lie and tell you I've never thought about the dirty deed of suicide. The thought is there, like a big bonfire that I'm dancing around. When will I jump in? My mother did when I was twenty-six. My grandfather did when I was four or five. Personally, I know at least a dozen guys who have done it, died by suicide—the final option to cure the pain. Stop the hurt and the fear of missing out.

I always imagined retiring to a life of surfing, skydiving, running, and swimming to my heart's delight. All those things that I love... a lot of my friends still do, but I can't do anymore because my body is racked. My feet and knees are in terrible condition. My shoulders can't take the repetitive strokes of swimming. And my back, which I broke in the early 90s, is only getting worse. Depression sets in even more when I ruminate over the fact that I can no longer do any of these activities.

My relationship with my two biological daughters from my first marriage is less than optimal, to put it mildly. Coping with all of this is draining and requires energy and compartmentalizing, putting these "things" into boxes and shelving each one as best I can.

Sometimes these boxes fall off the shelf and expose all the emotions that must be dealt with. So, how do I deal with all of it these days? I look for new ways and techniques to work out. I exercise with very deliberate intentions. I can no longer just head out the door for an exhilarating run or go swim a mile to clear my head. Weights are lifted in a certain way to avoid exacerbating an old injury. This means no dynamic style exercising.

Managing depression and the "ultimate side effect" is a daily thing for me. It requires me to think and act in specific ways and with a sense of purpose, shedding how I used to think. Getting upset over the small stuff, things out of my control is unnecessary. No more rants of negativity. Old feelings over people need to be discarded in order to get my head straight. In some cases, this means forgiving people for perceived sins against me. I am making sure I take the prescribed medications to alleviate the physical pain and discomfort my old profession left me with: neuropathy, chronic pain in almost every joint, and depression. With the help of my therapist, I better manage everything (from my brain to my feet) more than ever before. I guess that's what getting old is—managing all the pain. I'm only sixty years old, but some days it feels older—dog years, I guess. I have to cut myself some slack for the bad memory and be okay with the sticky notes that litter my desk.

It's not easy some days. Those are the days I dance around the fire.

# MEET STEVE GIBLIN

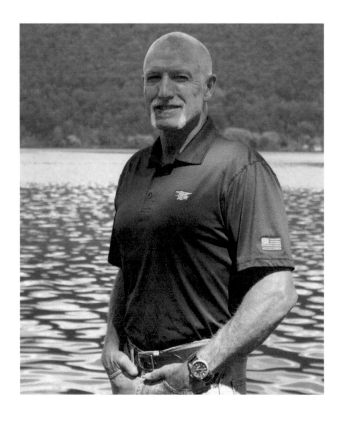

Steve Giblin, a retired Navy SEAL, embodies the essence of dedication, discipline, and resilience. Born and raised with an unwavering commitment to service, Steve's journey led him through the ranks of the US Navy SEALs, where he honed his skills in the crucible of adversity.

During his military career, Steve undertook numerous assignments and positions, displaying steadfast followership and leadership and an indomitable spirit. Determined towards commitment and leadership, he became a symbol of what most would imagine, a Master Chief you didn't want to cross, but also had your six when backed into a corner.

Transitioning to civilian life, Steve and his wife found solace in the tranquil landscapes of the Southwest. Embracing the challenges of retirement, he remained an active advocate for Veteran support programs and community.

In the arid beauty of the Southwest, Steve discovered a new mission – fostering resilience in his fellow man through writing and camaraderie with fellow teammates. Today, his legacy extends beyond the battlefield as he continues to uplift others, embodying the SEAL ethos in the heart of the desert.

∾

**Connect with Steve**
**Navy SEAL Master Chief (Ret.)**

*Author of Walking in Mud: A Navy SEAL's 10 Rules for Surviving the New Normal*

*LinkedIn: Steve Giblin*

∾

# Your Turn

What came up for you in this story?

_____
_____
_____
_____
_____
_____
_____
_____
_____
_____
_____
_____
_____
_____
_____
_____
_____
_____
_____
_____
_____
_____
_____
_____
_____

# CHAPTER 5
## COMING HOME

*by*
*Shad Meshad*

A psychiatric social worker, I went to Nam by choice. It was the first time the military had deployed mental health teams in a combat zone. We were a team of fifteen serving 500,000. Besides the wild beauty and the humidity, what impressed me on my arrival was the long line of dead-eyed troops filing out to the plane we'd just landed in. A year later, I was one of them. Nixon's early drop to be home for Christmas.

When we landed at Travis AFB, an officer came aboard and told us we had to clear customs before being bussed out to the processing center. We gathered our gear and filed down the ramp to the waiting customs lines. As I got near, I saw some of the troops were being led away in handcuffs. The MPs grabbed one of the troops, threw him down and handcuffed him. Then they picked him up and hurried him away.

I was really wired and was shaking by the time I reached the front of the line. The agent looked at my bars and said, "Okay, Captain, you can go through."

"What's going on with those troops who were handcuffed?"

"They were busted for drugs, Captain. They think they're pretty sharp, that just because they were over there, they can bring anything they want in here. They sell it when they get here. We're on 'em as soon as they get here."

"Check my bag," I told him.

"You're okay," he told me, waving me through.

"I said, check my fucking bag," I screamed. I was ready to hit somebody.

The confused agent grabbed my bags and gave them a perfunctory check.

A couple of black troops had been behind me in line and on the plane. They came up behind me and asked if I was crazy, fucking with the guy like that.

"That asshole can check my bags like anybody else's," I exploded. "I'm tired of the officers being separated from all the shit. What about those poor guys getting busted? What kind of homecoming is that?"

I boarded the bus heading to Oakland base. As we approached the Oakland entrance, we saw hundreds of students carrying signs ranging from baby-killer slogans to End the War. Bottles and bricks this time. As stones and Molotov cocktails broke against the sides of our bus, some of the troops instinctively dove. The students were young Americans. Many were our age.

I was furious and trying to see their faces to remember them.

One black troop asked me if I was a doctor, and I told him sort of and asked him what he was.

"Just a dumb fucking grunt like the others on this bus. But I made it back, doc. I made it back. What do you think is going on? Do you think we're gonna have trouble or something?"

We started assuring each other it was just Oakland. The rest of the country would not be like that. We loosened up.

At Oakland, we were told that processing would begin at five the following morning, December 23rd. Officers and enlisted men were separated and sent to barracks.

I couldn't get the homecoming scene out of my mind. Those troops being busted and their bags torn into. The whole system was unfair to enlisted men, not only over there, but here too. I had freaked out in customs, but I was proud of it.

The way the men were being treated was incredible. I kept thinking people didn't know what they were dealing with. Deep down, every troop who de-boarded that plane was a time bomb. No one seemed to heed that or care.

When I completed my processing out the next morning, I called an old and dear friend from Alabama who was living near San Francisco. The day before had really shaken me up. I was wired, angry, shaky, and coming unraveled. She could see I was in no condition to get on a plane and arrive at my parents' door, but I wouldn't let her talk me into staying. Through friends, she maneuvered a ticket home for me. I didn't even want her to come into the airport with me.

Most troops had been waiting a few days to get on standby. They had no contacts. Would they ever get home? The airport was in shock. GIs everywhere—lying on the floors, standing and sitting by the counters, propped up in deep sleep against their duffle bags and the walls. Some paced back and forth like tigers in a cage. Vietnam was all over them. I was in slow motion, walking toward the ticket counter, stepping over all the soldiers with confusion in their eyes. It was like being back in Danang.

I heard screaming and walked in that direction. One of the troops, a black guy, came running up to me when he saw my captain's bars and said to me, "Captain, you won't believe this. They got us a Christmas drop, and now there ain't no airplanes to get us home. And they're checking us out to see if we have alcohol on our breath. If we do, they won't let us fly."

He pointed at three brothers arguing with a blonde agent at the counter. She was screaming at them, and they were just standing there as if they were being talked down to by their commanding officer.

"If you come back up to the counter, I'm going to call the police," she screamed. "I told you, you will not get on the next plane, whether or not you have your tickets because you are all inebriated."

One started to plead with her, putting out his hands. They had been waiting at the airport three days, he told her. They stood there, all three of them taking turns begging her.

I put down my bags and ran up to the counter and got in front of the troops, so I could get right up in her face.

"Look, bitch," I said, "these sons of bitches have been fighting a war, so you can sit here and have your job and work and live in this land that gives you your freedom. They've been out there pounding in the bush, and you're gonna say they can't get in a plane to head home, when they haven't been there in a year, because they're inebriated?"

She began screaming at me now, her face incredibly red, threatening to call the police on me too.

"Call them!" I shouted.

A crowd was gathering around the counter, and a manager came running across the floor. I jumped up on the counter and yelled at the agent, "Who are you to pull regulations on them? They've had regulations pulled on them for two years or more. They want to go home!"

I wanted to mash her. I wanted to pick her up by her blonde hair and throw her to the troops. Instead, I sweated and pounded and stomped my foot on the counter. I was so hysterical I didn't know what I was saying.

Airport security came, and two officers began grabbing my legs. The manager began pleading with me to get down. Meanwhile the girl is crying and sobbing, and I'm yelling at her,

"That's right. Cry all you want. You don't know what it's like to die and bleed over there, do you?"

I jumped down before they had to pull me down, and the manager asked the police to bring me to his office, saying he could handle everything.

I was totally in the war, waging a battle, my senses locked full on, fueled by an uncontrollable, hysterical rage. The manager's office filled with police and airport security. He just asked me to relax for a minute, and he had the three troops brought in. They came in looking shocked, certain they were in trouble.

"I want these three men given top priority, and I want them put on the plane first. I want them to be given anything they want until they reach their destination," he told someone at the door.

He asked to see my tickets, and I gave them to him.

"I want him escorted down to the right gate," he said.

Someone had me by the arm and was walking with me through the boarding area. I didn't even look at the person. The three brothers came over, hugged me and thanked me, and I hardly noticed.

I waded through the green uniforms, heading for my gate, and felt hands slapping me on the back. But something had shifted in that blind rage as I stood on the counter yelling at that ticket agent. The fire of the injustice and the mindlessness of the treatment being dealt to those combat vets coming home lit me up. I was outraged, but it sparked a determination to make a difference that has lasted over fifty years. It was going to be harder than I thought, this coming home. Vietnam was coming with me. That rage changed my life and determined its direction as a lifelong advocate for Veterans.

I arrived home and like many others, I felt alienated from my country, friends and even my family. My father wept when I left Birmingham to drive across the country in a van outfitted as a camper for me and my girl. He knew I had to go. My only plan was to visit one of the sergeants I served with at the 95th Medical Evac Hospital in 'Nam. He'd gone back to LA to finish his education at USC. He dragged me along to a lecture, and that's how I met the head of the VA Hospital in Brentwood. It was the largest psychiatric hospital in the country. He needed to know why Vietnam vets were not using the VA. I was fresh back from 'Nam. He offered me a job. I declined. He was persistent and weeks later I finally agreed to take it on for ninety days.

To talk to Vets, I first had to find them. They're still in the same places: under bridges, camped out along dry riverbeds, in canyons, in abandoned buildings and even on a condemned pier. At first it was just conversation, then it was small groups. We got together and rapped. All over the city. I took what I'd learned back to the VA and was hired to run the first Vietnam Veterans Rehabilitation Unit in Westwood, LA.

In 1975, Max Cleland, a triple amputee who served as head of the VA, came to LA to check out the "Mad Man" as I was known. I pushed his chair all over Venice and the grounds of the VA hospital where medicated vets lounged in the sun. He understood what we were facing. Cleland wept and said, "That's the future for these guys if we don't do something big."

We did something big. He and Senator Alan Cranston invited me to Washington where I met President Carter. I'd come to Washington with Bill Mahedy, also a Vietnam vet who was a Veterans Service Officer. We did an all-nighter in October of 1977 in Washington, D.C., designing what is today the Vet

Center program. Later, Bill served as a counselor in the program Carter signed into law in 1979.

Fast forward. There are now over three-hundred Vet Centers in the country, all using the model of vet-to-vet counseling I developed in the streets of LA. In 1986, I left the VA's bureaucracy to establish what became the National Veterans Foundation to focus on real help in real time for Veterans. We opened the first national toll-free hotline to deliver information and resources to Vets. Later, we expanded our audience to include *all* Veterans and their families. We've run our Lifeline for Vets for over thirty-eight years and added a Street Outreach for homeless vets and an outreach for women Veterans. During the wars in Iraq and Afghanistan, the Lifeline even received calls from combat zones.

I've never forgotten the outrage I felt standing on the counter in that airport. I can feel the energy of it course through my body still, after fifty-three years of advocacy. It continues to power the National Veterans Foundation, now in its 39th year. There are times when you are pressed to the wall in a way that threatens to break you, but in fact, it can break into something way larger.

# MEET FLOYD "SHAD" MESHAD

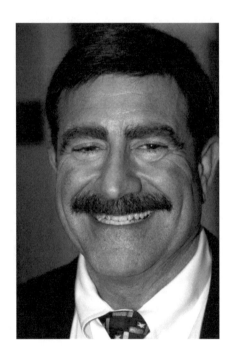

For over 52 years, Floyd "Shad" Meshad has been a therapist and advocate for Veterans' rights. He holds an MSW in psychiatric social work from Florida State University. He served as a psych officer in Vietnam, continuing to counsel VN Vets on the streets of LA. In 1985, he founded the National Veterans Foundation. It is now in its 39th year of service to Veterans and their families. The NVF's Lifeline for Vets was the first national toll-free number for Veterans' resources and crisis counseling.

Among the first to study and identify PTSD, Meshad co-authored the Vet Center Program, using his vet-to-vet counseling model. He opened the first locations, which now number over 300 nationwide.

He has served on the faculty of the International Critical Incident Stress Foundation, as president of the Association of Traumatic Stress Specialists and on the board of directors of the Green Cross Project.

A new edition of his 1982 Vietnam memoir, *Captain for Dark Mornings*, was republished in 2023 and is available in print, e-book and audiobook. In November of 2023, Meshad was inducted into the US Veterans Hall of Fame.

∼

### Connect with Shad

**US Army Captain, Medical Service Corps**

**Co-author of the Vet Center Program**

**President and Founder of the National Veterans Foundation**

**Author of Captain for Dark Mornings: Hidden Struggles Behind the Vietnam War**

*Email: shad@nvf.org*
*LinkedIn: Floyd 'Shad' Meshad*
*Website: www.nvf.org*

∼

# Your Turn

What came up for you in this story?

_____
_____
_____
_____
_____
_____
_____
_____
_____
_____
_____
_____
_____
_____
_____
_____
_____
_____
_____
_____
_____
_____
_____
_____
_____
_____
_____

# CHAPTER 6
# THE JOURNEY BACK TO TRUE EMPOWERMENT

*by*

*Michelle Franklin*

When you become a 911 dispatcher, you are taught that you're the center of everything. You're the key component to making everything run as smoothly as possible. Officer needs help? That's on you to know exactly where to send the help and what type of help to send. A parent calls 911 because their child is not breathing? It's on you to know how to get help started and provide the best life-saving measures possible.

I was a dispatcher for fourteen years; half of that time was spent as a supervisor. I worked for three different departments, all of which had the call sign "control" to get dispatch on the radio. That call sign, in and of itself, solidified that *I* was in control. I had the power, or so I thought.

This is my journey to finding my way back to true empowerment.

~

On January 7, 2021, I walked out of my communications center for the last time. Just to be clear, that was not my intention. My intention was to take some vacation time for the rest of the month and return refreshed and "back to normal." I was struggling with processing a very traumatic incident I worked on in November of 2020. My department placed a total of three dispatchers and approximately seventeen officers on paid administrative leave following that incident. They required each of us to see a psychiatrist and be cleared before returning to work. I was out for three weeks. It didn't help. I just wanted to get back to work, get back to "normal," so I just said whatever I needed to say so that the psychiatrist would clear me.

For the next month and a half, I struggled a lot. I was trying my best to push through each workday, but I was not holding myself to my typical high standard work ethic. I was very irritable when I talked to people, but mostly, I was withdrawn. I used up quite a bit of my sick leave. I'd call out for whole shifts, and when I did go to work, I usually left early. Sleeping was tough for me. I wasn't getting good sleep because of the nightmares. I was constantly picking fights with my boyfriend and snapping at my daughter without even realizing it.

It took a fellow dispatch supervisor to recognize my struggle. It was on that day (January 7, 2020) that she told me I needed to talk to our manager and take some time off or she was going to say something herself. Even in that moment, I still felt like I was in "control." I figured I could just take a few weeks off and get back to "normal." Unfortunately, instead of getting better, I got worse. Anxiety, paired with hyper-vigilance, became a controlling factor in my life. I'd limit going outside of my house because public spaces left me feeling out of control. I'd get anxiety attacks. A lot of times I would find myself paralyzed with fear. I'd just stay home, safe on my couch, as much as I could. This quickly led to me not getting dressed, which led to not showering or even brushing my hair. I wasn't eating enough, so I began losing weight. I couldn't track conversations. I'd forget what I was saying halfway through sentences. I was taking online classes to complete my bachelor's degree in psychology and ended up taking a medical leave because I had no ability to concentrate. I'd read an article for class and had no idea what I had just read. I was easily triggered by sounds, and there was a constant white noise in my head.

Flashbacks were a new normal for me. I sunk into a depression, which made it very difficult to care for my three-and-a-half-year-old daughter. I felt awful that she had to see me this way, but there was nothing I could do about it. My false sense of control was gone, and this was me crumbling. I tried to hide it for so long, but my brain was telling me it couldn't take anymore.

While being stuck in this darkness, I started the process for Workers' Compensation, since I was formally diagnosed with Post Traumatic Stress Disorder (PTSD). The case was accepted, and I started seeing a psychiatrist and a therapist. My therapist was a great fit for me. She was culturally competent and understood why certain things really bothered me. It is really important to find a therapist that fits you. I worked with plenty who were not the right fit, and it caused me some setbacks.

One day, a friend told me about this group of First Responders and Veterans who meet for virtual coffee and conversation every week. This group is called The Power of Our Story. My friend told me to check it out because she felt it would help me. I took the information and let it sit for a bit. I didn't feel like "socializing," even if it was only virtually. I definitely was not up for putting on my happy face. I think it was almost a month before I decided to give it a shot. I jumped on one night and heard the story of one of the most amazing people I know. His name is Aaron Terrill. He shared his journey with Traumatic Brain Injury (TBI), PTSD and other medical conditions caused by an injury while on duty as a police officer.

Now, allow me to explain something. The traumatic incident I worked on back in November of 2020 cut through to the very core of who I am. It  shocked my soul. This is how deeply it affected me. It was the icing on the cake, the reason for my mental shut down and entrance into a storm of darkness. Almost one year later, I heard Aaron's story for the first time. It was like electricity to my soul. It gave me the shock I needed to begin my fight out of the darkness. He was able to put into words all the craziness and emotions I was feeling. He was able to explain what I couldn't find the words to voice. He understood me even though he had never met me. His vulnerability that night showed me that I wasn't alone. There was a small beam of light starting to show through my storm.

I started regularly attending The Power of Our Story. I started off silent, never saying much. Just listening. Slowly, as I grew more comfortable, I started to speak about my own experiences and struggles. This group of people became genuine friends, never judging me, and offering support and advice. I needed this. This group became a pillar on my journey of healing.

It was through The Power of Our Story that I found resources to help me, like a sleep program called 62Romeo. I am getting a good night's sleep again. 22Zero was also a resource that helped me process a lot of other traumatic incidents. It was all just one Zoom call away. I am forever grateful to Sara Correll, the founder of The Power of Our Story. The virtual platform she created for those of us suffering in silence is so needed. In that way, COVID-19 became a blessing. That was exactly what I needed because, at the time, there was no way I was leaving my house, especially to go to a public place, meet a group of strangers, and talk about the deepest, most vulnerable parts of myself ... not in the state I was in. I am forever grateful.

I have since settled my workers' compensation case, and my family and I have moved to another state. We live in a smaller city with a slower pace of life. It has been the perfect fit for me, as I continue my mental health journey. I currently work at a university where my value is based on me as a person and not what I do for the organization. I enrolled in school and completed my bachelor's degree and have since started on my master's. I have started Eye Movement Desensitization and Reprocessing therapy (EMDR), and it has really helped me turn flashbacks into memories, so I am not crippled by them when they creep into my mind.

The biggest success for me is that I've found my power. More importantly, after living fourteen years with a false sense of control, I discovered the truth about my power. Now, I know that my power is the ability to ask for help when I am struggling. My power is taking time off from work for mental health's sake, to attend my EMDR sessions. My power is in finding my own identity versus associating it with what I do for a living. My power is in being vulnerable and sharing my story so that others can know they are not alone. The journey was tough. I'd even venture to say it may be one of the hardest roads I've taken. But once the light returned and all the pieces fell into place, that hard road was worth it! I do not wish my trauma on anyone, nor do I wish to repeat it. However, it has gotten me to where I am today, and for that, I am grateful!

# MEET MICHELLE FRANKLIN

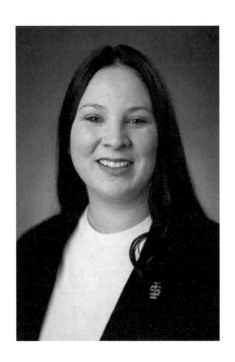

Michelle Franklin spent 14 years as a 911 dispatcher and supervisor. In 2020, life created a perfect storm which left her with a diagnosis of Post-Traumatic Stress Disorder (PTSD) and the loss of her career. Through her journey of healing, Michelle is learning the true meaning of empowerment. She has shifted her career and is now happily working at Idaho State University. She is also serving as the social media coordinator for The Power of Our Story, a platform that invites Veterans and First

Responders into a safe space, where they soon discover they do not need to suffer in silence.

Michelle is happily engaged to her fiancé, Kyle. They have three children. When she is not working or spending time with her family, she is studying to complete a master's degree in public administration.

### Connect with Michelle
#### 911 Dispatcher Supervisor (Ret.)

*LinkedIn: Michelle Franklin*

# Your Turn

What came up for you in this story?

_____
_____
_____
_____
_____
_____
_____
_____
_____
_____
_____
_____
_____
_____
_____
_____
_____
_____
_____
_____
_____
_____
_____
_____
_____
_____
_____
_____

# CHAPTER 7
# THE DAY CURIOSITY SAVED
# MY LIFE

*By*
*Michael Halterman*

I lose one Veteran, someone I know personally, every year to suicide. As my network increases outside of the Veteran community, I also lose one or two civilian friends to suicide every year. With some of my Veteran friends, you can almost see it coming. They have tough childhoods, so they join the military, looking for identity, community, purpose, and meaning. They find it, especially in Special Operations. They train and deploy to combat zones at a much higher rate than the norm. Then, at some point, they leave active-duty service and are stripped of their identity, community, purpose, and meaning. This, coupled with all the unresolved trauma, leaves them feeling isolated and vulnerable. You can literally watch their lives spiral with a cascade of bad decisions, like joining biker gangs and drug use. Others, however, demonstrate no outward indicator. They are involved in life and community and have loving mothers and fathers. In either case, there is generally a phone call or text message that follows, sharing that they are gone.

My story is not so different. It was a beautiful day. I was standing in my backyard. The sky was blue and clear—big, white, billowy clouds in the sky. I could see all the way to the mountains. I was in a very positive mood before walking outside. I was thinking about completing projects at work and what I would be having for dinner that evening, and then, literally, out of nowhere, it struck me ... I should end my life.

I didn't have bad things going on in my life. I wasn't ruminating on how bad things were. I wasn't in chronic pain. I did not just go through a traumatic event, but the idea of ending my life hit me like a force. The only way I can describe it is to say that it was like being possessed by a spirit. I was fully gripped by it. It was more than just a thought or an idea; it was a sheer force of will, and it fully engulfed me. I knew without a doubt that was what I had to do next. There was no fear or sadness. I just knew it was what I had to do. There was, however, a momentary hesitation because I got curious. I got curious about where this thought could possibly be coming from. Was it outside of me? Was it inside of me? Where did it come from? How did it get in ... and so forcefully? Why was I totally happy one minute, enjoying the day, going from everything is fine to completely and totally possessed by this idea, this spirit telling me that I should end my life?

Instead of pushing the thought away, trying to fight it, becoming afraid of it, pondering if I had done something wrong or if my life was that bad, I just continued to be curious and ask myself questions, things like "Is this what happens to my Veteran brothers and sisters?" "Does it fully engulf their thoughts like it had mine, and is there no one to help them if it does?"

I thought, perhaps, if those thoughts hit them when they are most vulnerable, all the negative emotion just adds to their resolve to end their life. There is no pause for curiosity. Because of my experience, I think suicide is like cancer. It is in almost all of us, and some of us die from it. The rest of us die with it still in us. I got lucky.

Having such a visceral and personal brush with suicide, matched with my experience with war, leads me to believe that everyone is suffering and hurting in ways we cannot even imagine. That is why I try to be patient, understanding, and love anyone who steps in front of me and interacts with me. I try to be curious about others and see if I can help them. If, through even just a simple smile, I can alleviate their suffering for a moment, I will do just that. To date, I've helped more than a few individuals while they're struggling with suicidal thoughts, perhaps even more who I did not know were struggling. Curiosity saved my life. Now, I try to be more focused and intentional about my curiosity because I see it as a superpower that I can use to help others.

# MEET MICHAEL HALTERMAN

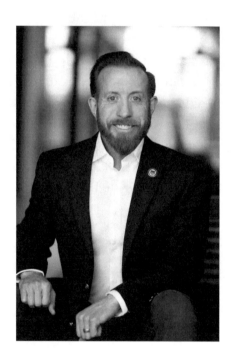

*"I solve the problems of tomorrow so others can bridge to the future."*

Michael Halterman was born and raised in a small town on the Central Coast of California. Growing up, he played multiple team sports and loved to skateboard. In high school, he worked multiple construction labor jobs and food service positions. During the crush season, he also worked in the vineyards and cellars of wineries.

From 1998 to 2006, Michael was an infantryman in the United States Marine Corps. He deployed overseas four times, including one invasion in Iraq in 2003. From 2007 to his military retirement in 2018, Michael served as a Marine Raider in Special Operations. He deployed four more times, three of which were to Afghanistan. Upon transition from active-duty military service, Michael joined The Honor Foundation (THF) to help other Special Operations Veterans transition. Michael started his career at The Honor Foundation as the first director of Virtual Programs. Michael is now the vice president of Operations, overseeing all back-office operations. When he is not at work, he can be found hiking, camping, rock climbing, and mountaineering.

∽

**Connect with Michael**
*Marine Raider (Ret.)*

*LinkedIn: Michael G. Halterman*

∽

# Your Turn

What came up for you in this story?

_____
_____
_____
_____
_____
_____
_____
_____
_____
_____
_____
_____
_____
_____
_____
_____
_____
_____
_____
_____
_____
_____
_____
_____
_____
_____

# CHAPTER 8
# THAT OTHERS MAY LIVE

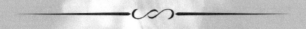

*By*

*Glenn Ignazio*

In the Air Force Special Operations community, we have a persona of being "The Quiet Professionals." Therefore, many may not be familiar with our missions. Air Force Special Operations infiltrate and exfiltrate teams, such as the SEALs, Green Berets, and "Others" to get in and out of their mission areas, anywhere in the world. Additionally, we conduct combat rescue of those in harm's way. This means we get "Special Teams," pilots who have been shot down and "Other" customers out of bad situations behind enemy lines. In combat rescue, we perform extremely dangerous missions that others can't or won't. When our missions fail, the result is grim. Yet, we press on because we know that we are all that remain for those in dire straits. You quickly learn; it is easy to embrace success. It is much harder to embrace failure. Even though the knowledge you gain and the character you build is so powerful, you never forget the missions you failed—it's a hard pill to swallow.

I'll never forget that night. We were alerted to a life and death mission. We immediately scrambled to the aircraft, ready to press. As we taxied to the runway, the weather was horrific. Not only was it a night operation, but there was a sandstorm— visibility was terrible for both take-off and landing.

An Army helicopter (Helo) was airborne, performing mission rehearsals before the beginning of the war. Flying around the desert, day or night, is tricky. The situation was sudden and violent. The Blackhawk helicopter was flying up to 130 knots under night vision, operating as low as possible. Unfortunately, a tank berm went unseen, and the helicopter struck it. This caused the Blackhawk to crash into flames. We had various airborne surveillance assets, allowing us to see the crash and what was happening in real-time.

I was on the runway, throttles ready to push up for takeoff. The Blackhawk crew was less than twenty miles away, a ten-minute flight to save these warriors. The surveillance resource could see the aircraft burning; soldiers were alive. Someone was crawling away from the wreckage. I cannot describe the emotions. I'm a visual person. I could picture the scene, a soldier critically injured on the desert floor in pitch black, the only light coming from the flames of his burning aircraft. Having just experienced a horrific crash and losing crew members, he was all alone. It was that image and one warrior's desperation that moved me to do everything in my power to save him. My crew and I sensed the deteriorating situation. It's what drives us to do what we do. It's my personal contract and commitment to risk my life to save another. However, with all the emotions, I must maintain balance so as not to kill my own crew. Pure discipline separates emotion from logic. Sounds easy in text, but it is a monumental task in real life.

The sandstorm was so bad that I could barely see the lines on the runway. We just wanted to take off and get there. Self-preservation was not a thought. However, the discipline compels intelligence, logic, and wisdom in what we do. Every emotion was screaming, "GO!" Logic responded, "STOP!"

I cannot describe the feeling in words, sitting on a runway, throttle in hand, ready to hurl into the desolate, dark void to save a brother or sister in arms who, quite possibly, could be experiencing their last moments on Earth. I had to make the conscious decision **not** to do anything because it could mean more American souls dying on the desert floor. The feeling was horrible. Imagine being feet away from a friend or family member, watching them perish as you must sit there and do nothing but watch. That trauma never leaves you—ever!

You torment yourself afterwards, contemplating what you could have done. I could have held there, waiting for the weather to clear or even a lull in the storm that would allow us to take off. It was our commitment: *These things we do, that others may live.* That's when we heard the nightmare radio call. There was no more movement on that dark desert floor—he died alone. The inability to complete a mission is emotional. However, I could not cave into those feelings. I had to recover quickly since I was still on alert, but it was difficult to process and carry knowing that fellow warriors perished on my watch. Saving them was my mission. It was why I existed in that dark desert!

There was no way an event like this was not going to have a negative impact on my mental health, and this was only one of many missions in my career. I could choose to deal with it or bury it. If burying it only makes it bigger, how much can one warrior bury before opening up, or worse, breaking? I wondered; was I the only one feeling this way? Would others criticize me for feeling this way? This is the challenge with PTSD in the military.

It was difficult for me to open up because I believed flight surgeons would ground me or I would be judged by others.

So, I compartmentalized the event, suppressing my thoughts and pressing on with the next mission at hand. Not a great long-term plan, since suppression surfaced sixteen years later, when I was introduced to a wonderful lady at a birthday party in her home. I saw her son's uniform framed and hanging on the wall. I asked her where he was stationed; she told me that he died in Iraq. Overwhelming emotions surged; vivid images raced through my mind as if it was happening at that moment. Was he one of the Blackhawk crew? Was I in the presence of a Gold Star Mother whose son was lost on the mission I couldn't complete? Was I responsible? I excused myself, then broke into tears in the bathroom. As it turned out, her son was not one of those men, but it was no less difficult to absolve. I needed help. It was not comfortable opening up and discussing these feelings. I thought less of myself, until someone said, "It's not that you are not strong; it's that you have been strong too long."

I wish I had opened up sooner. I am opening up now by sharing my story to help others in similar situations. Getting help is not a judgement on your character, nor is it failure. Both are a powerful tool, teaching you and motivating you to go further than you ever have before. Failure is not something to fear; it's an important lesson to carry forward.

Flying for Special Operations and combat rescue has been an incredible journey, which taught me about the value of life. I had my challenges and failures, not just on these missions but in a high-altitude accident that ended my career and almost took my life. I had a decompression accident at 35,000 feet. The damage was bad enough to pull me out of the cockpit, ending my service in the Air Force and requiring numerous surgeries. I have more metal parts in me now than I ever expected.

The sudden transition out of uniform was a significant

challenge, more difficult than some may understand. One day I was flying a multi-million-dollar aircraft with people's lives in my hands, and the next day I was unemployed. The feeling of isolation and uncertainty was overbearing. When I was injured, I spent three days in the hospital at Travis Air Force Base. When I was not in a hyperbaric chamber, I was alone in a hospital room, in the wing for those injured in Iraq and Afghanistan. Except for me, there were no other patients. I was isolated, and I didn't realize the negative impact on me until years later. During my stay, I only heard from two people in my unit and that was only because we were good friends. No commanders or flight leads could be bothered to visit or check on me. I laid there, feeling abandoned, wondering what was happening to me and my future.

I had multiple surgeries that spanned two years, ending my civilian career and impacting my life in Silicon Valley. In a few short years, I lost my career, my health, my hobbies, my purpose, my marriage, my home, and even my dog. It sounds like a bad country song, but it was real. There have been more than a few unexpected challenges.

For one, I had never used narcotics, but suddenly I was on pain killers to manage the hellish pain. I avoided medication in the military. So, I went from zero to 240mg of pure oxycodone a day for twenty-two months. I became addicted; there was no way I couldn't be. I had to go through a program to get off the pain killers. I was embarrassed and ashamed, regardless of it being prescribed. To my surprise, the program had members from different career fields, including Special Forces. I was the only officer and pilot. Right then and there, I changed my mindset, and I did what I had to do. I was determined not to quit. I didn't give up on myself or the other members of the program. I led by example and became a mentor, because I understood how dark the trauma can get.

My changing moment was seeing the physical and mental relief in the eyes of a distraught, enlisted soldier who had beaten himself up so badly for being addicted to narcotics. When he learned that I, an officer and pilot, understood and was in a similar place, he went easier on himself. I felt that I may have saved him from a possible suicide. My newfound purpose (mission) is to help people, military and civilian, get up after getting knocked down. I want people to know that they are not alone. It is a way I can continue to save myself and others—a rescue mission, only less dangerous.

# MEET GLENN IGNAZIO

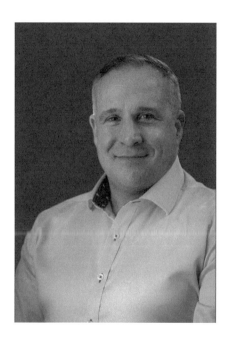

Glenn Ignazio is a Retired Air Force Special Operations Pilot, National Security Advisor and Defense Intelligence Technology expert. His experience has made him a sought-after national security, geo-political advisor and media contributor. He is active on US and international news networks, such as News Nation, CNN, NewsMax, Fox News, Sky News and the Canadian TV network.

Glenn has conducted numerous rescues, in and out of service, including the negotiated hostage release of a senior executive in the Middle East. He is highly decorated with Single Mission Air Medals, Air Force Commendation Medals, and Special Operations Citations. He also received United States Congressional Recognition for Combat Operations.

Following his military service, Glenn continues to provide aid in hostile environments, including establishing evacuation operations for civilians trapped within combat areas in the Russian-Ukraine conflict. He coordinated the evacuation of American citizens, civilians, and friendly forces during the hasty withdrawal from Afghanistan.

Glenn continues to be a champion for Veterans, speaking on the topics of PTSD and addiction recovery, as well as the prevention of Veteran suicide. He is a keynote speaker on the personal ethic of Failing Forward; not giving in but rather getting up when faced with overwhelming odds.

∿

### *Connect with Glenn*
*Combat Rescue and Special Operations Pilot, Major USAF (Ret.)*

*LinkedIn: Glenn Ignazio*
*Facebook: Glenn Ignazio*
*Instagram: Glenn.Ignazio*
*Website: www.Glenn-Ignazio.com*

∿

# Your Turn

What came up for you in this story?

_____

_____

_____

_____

_____

_____

_____

_____

_____

_____

_____

_____

_____

_____

_____

_____

_____

_____

_____

_____

_____

_____

_____

# CHAPTER 9

# TWO VALLEYS AND A SUMMIT —HOW PAINFUL JOURNEYS CAN FORGE BEAUTIFUL ANSWERS

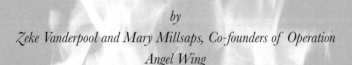

*by*
*Zeke Vanderpool and Mary Millsaps, Co-founders of Operation Angel Wing*

**M**y valley approached rock bottom as I walked across a beautiful Eastern Kentucky hillside in late spring of 2003. Crickets sang. The branches of old, magnificent hardwood trees that stood watch over our family cemetery swayed gently in the breeze under a soft blue sky.

I made my way through the vestiges of what was left behind by generations of my family, their names etched in stone with dates that spanned from the 1800's until the most recent—August 2002. That one belonged to my mother.

Mom died two weeks before I deployed to Afghanistan.

In New York City, they were still picking body parts out of the rubble of the twin towers. At Fort McClellan, Alabama, my military unit, 20th Special Forces Group, was frantically preparing to deploy and replace the current Special Forces Group on the ground in northern Afghanistan. In Knoxville, Tennessee, my mother was very sick. My reality seemed to fit, in lockstep, with the chaos that our Country was experiencing.

I got the call right after I finished a "shoot on the move" training iteration on Pellham range. The heat index every day that week was over one-hundred-ten degrees and there was no shade on the firing range. "Go to war" rules were in effect. There was no cancelling training due to danger of heat injuries. If someone went down, the medic pushed an IV, rehydrated them, and it was back to work. As I was reloading mags and pounding water, dad called. His voice broke as he told me the news. "Son, your mom is in bad shape. She's at Saint Mary's in the ICU. They don't expect her to last more than a few days."

I sat beside my mom's bed for three days. I held her hand and talked to her. I read to her. I just tried to be present with her. Though she never regained consciousness, she would squeeze my hand and her heart rate would increase when I spoke. It was the most precious time that I ever spent with my mother. And then she was gone. Two weeks later, I climbed on a big bird, flew to the other side of the planet, and landed in the hornet's nest known as Afghanistan.

Funny thing about a combat zone—it's more than likely one of the most dangerous places you will ever experience (depending on your hobbies and dating preferences, of course), but if you survive it, and most people do, you will come to realize it as a place where you felt more alive, connected, and focused than any other time in your life. Unfortunately, this dynamic can work both for the better and the worse. Throughout that year I spent in Afghanistan, a lot happened in my head and in my heart. I thought I had it covered. I learned I could build a box deep in my mind, and I could shove pain (both physical and emotional) into that box. It was amazing how much I could pack into it. At the end of that year, in the back of my mind, I took sixteen-penny nails and a hammer, and I nailed that son of a bitch shut. Then I came home.

After several months of trying to fit back in as a husband, father, son, police officer, friend, and general member of my beloved community, I found myself failing miserably. Inwardly, I was in a state of turmoil and confusion and deep hurt that I had no language for. I could not articulate the fact that the only tribe I could connect to was the one I had gone to war with—those guys who, at least the ones who were still alive—had spread to the winds and gone back to their own families and, I would later learn, were experiencing the same shit storm that I was. Outwardly, I was steadily offending random people and family members. I was missing key moments as a dad, unapproachable as a husband, and mainly distant to those who knew me and were openly thankful that I was home. My responses and behavior just left them confused and concerned.

That brings us to a beautiful spring afternoon on an Eastern Kentucky hillside. Three very distinct things happened in rapid succession on that day, as I approached the foot of my mother's grave. First, a storm descended—violently. The sky transformed from a pastel blue to charcoal black almost instantaneously. Fat, warm drops of rain began to smack against my face like globs of spit from the heavens. The chirps of crickets and the gentle song of the breeze in the trees gave way to a roar of furious wind, seemingly bending the trees to their breaking point and ushering in a crazy, sideways curtain of rain that had turned cold and was now hitting like BB's.

The second thing that happened in that moment was even more surprising. The box that I had supposedly safely sealed shut months before in the back of my mind blew wide open. I dropped to my knees at the foot of my mother's grave, in the midst of the fury of that storm, and proceeded to come unglued at the seams of my soul. I wept. I wept for the loss of my mother, for the loss of my brothers in arms, for the loss of my identity, and for the innocence that somehow disappeared along with all of it. I cursed the reality that I was still alive and others I loved were not. I was furious at God and with the world and even more so with myself for being so weak. I screamed at the storm, and it screamed at me.

And then the third thing happened—maybe the most significant of everything that transpired on that day. Just as quickly as the storm had descended, it lifted. The sun pierced a hole in the dark clouds and scattered them almost instantly. The wind vanished and the trees stood upright again, water dripping on the grass below. The crickets picked up where they had left off. And there I sat on my knees at the foot of my mother's grave, not a dry stitch on my body. Little ponds had gathered in the indentations that my knees had made. I learned in that moment. The boxes don't work. At least, not for the long haul.

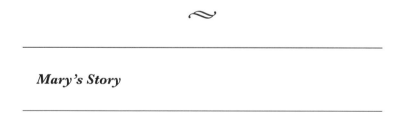

### Mary's Story

MARY'S VALLEY BOTTOMED OUT WHEN SHE WAS BEATEN unconscious and left for dead.

As a young woman in her early 20's, and after years of being married to a monster, she had finally decided that she could no longer live this way. She made the decision that the next time he decided to break her body, she would fight to the end. That's what she did; she went down swinging. With the beautiful but broken heart of a young woman who could take no more and the spirit of a true fighter, she answered his rage with her own.

He had beaten her so many times. He had kicked the unborn baby in her womb to death. He had followed her when she tried to run and dragged her home, each time with a high price. In her world there was no hope left. She sought the only peace that she could still connect to, that release that would wait for her on the other side of this battle, in her own death. So, on that day, she fought back. With everything in her.

He placed her unconscious, seemingly lifeless, broken frame across the foot of the bed and left to get his mother to come help him dispose of the evidence. It was a family of monsters. But in the moments that followed, something incredible happened. Mary awoke.

At first, she could not move. She only connected to the awareness that she was still alive. And with this dawning awareness came a new realization; she *wanted* to be alive. The faith that she had lost awakened with her. She tried to get up but fell to the floor. Her legs would not respond. So, she began to crawl, dragging herself to the kitchen and through the back door with the knowledge that upon his return she had no chance. She was able to get the attention of her neighbor, an elderly lady who immediately came to her. It was the last time he ever got his hands on her—Mary's story would continue.

From birth, it was a story that danced with demons and angels. Mary, a beautiful baby girl, was born to a depressed and addicted mother who abandoned her at birth. Mary's grandparents, a gentle and amazing World War II Veteran and his fiery, Irish wife—Maw and Paw—became her custodial parents, giving her an early reference of stability and love that she would later cling to when all else deserted her.

Mary's mother returned to her life, perpetuating horrific violence that a child should never know. As a thirteen-year-old girl, Mary was sexually trafficked by her sister and then held prisoner in a room by her mother. Her brother knew she would not survive the trauma and abuse, so he opened the door and set her free.

"You have to go …" he said.

Mary instantly became homeless, but she was alive. The owner of a diner, not asking any questions, gave that homeless girl a job, providing what he could … until Mary met the man who would manipulate, marry, and brutalize her, leaving her for dead.

If our stories are allowed to continue, despite the struggle, and we embrace them as a "journey," we *will* find that there is beauty and untold strength within. We can discover the divine power within our story to lead others through valleys when nothing else can. And within that gift, our own journey of healing continues.

AT THE LOW POINT IN OUR VALLEYS, MARY AND I DID NOT KNOW each other. We were simply trying to navigate our paths and move forward. I completed my military service, retiring in 2013 after my last combat tour in Iraq and continued in the field of Law Enforcement. Mary completed an amazing career in Emergency Medicine, retiring as an occupational healthcare administrator. She then earned her Master's in Neuro Linguistic Programming, emerging with an amazing ability to recognize and heal those struggling with the effects of trauma.

Then, in late 2013, our paths intersected. We compared notes and realized that we had the same mission in mind. Together, we co-founded Operation Angel Wing. We learned to use our life experience to connect to people of trauma when no one else could. We developed incredibly effective tools and approaches to heal them, healing our own wounds along the way. In the decade since, we have created an organization that shepherds people through the struggle and beyond, connecting them to purpose and forward motion. Our journeys through our own valleys came together, and from them we created an amazing summit.

~

## Quote from Mary Millsaps, Creator and Co-founder of Operation Angel Wing:

*"This mission comes from more than just my training and experience; it is the culmination of my life's work. As a young woman, I lived the reality of domestic violence. As a professional, I was and am a healer and protector. Through Operation Angel Wing, I am able to share the gift of finding a voice where I once had none and the power of healing and change in the presence of adversity."*

## Quote from Zeke Vanderpool, Co-founder of Operation Angel Wing:

*"My passion for Operation Angel Wing began with the struggle that occurs on the other side of war, behind closed doors, when the battlefield has become silent. Through my own challenges and those of my brothers and sisters around me, I knew that we had to find a better way to deal with traumatic stress. I am thankful every day for my partner and what we have created within this organization."*

~

# MEET ZEKE VANDERPOOL

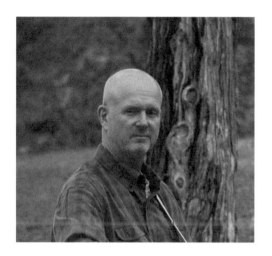

Zeke Vanderpool, Co-Founder, Chief Operations Officer and Coaching Team Lead of Operation Angel Wing, retired from the United States Army in 2013. With 23 years in Special Operations, he served in multiple theaters of operation, including Afghanistan and Iraq. As of 2024, he is finishing up a civilian career in Federal Law Enforcement, where he has served for over 20 years as a federal agent in defense and protection of our nation's Homeland Security.

Zeke attributes his greatest blessings to his relationship with God, his family, and the amazing people he has walked alongside in service of his country. As a singer-songwriter, he uses his life experience to connect to our nation's protectors, creating a foundation of trust and relevance that lead them to stronger and better ground. He continually seeks to make a positive impact on the lives of those who have given so much in the service of others.

∾

### Connect with Zeke
**Co-Founder, Chief Operations Officer and Coaching**

**Team Lead of Operation Angel Wing**

*Email: zeke@operationangelwing.org*
*Website: https://www.operationangelwing.org/*

∾

# MEET MARY MILLSAPS

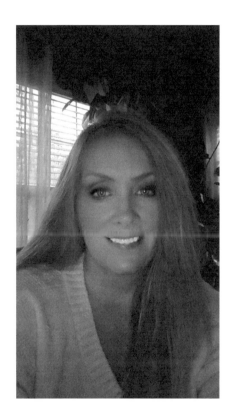

Mary Millsaps, creator and co-founder of Operation Angel Wing (OPAW), continually pours her life's work into pioneering innovative and effective ways to assist our Nation's men and women of service, their families, and the communities they serve —"One victory at a time."

Mary's personal struggle and succeeding dedication to her community led her to her calling and to the creation of OPAW. As a teen and young woman, she endured extreme and prolonged cycles of abuse. Despite her physical and emotional scars, she went on to complete a successful career in Emergency Medicine that spanned more than 20 years. She advanced from search and rescue to prehospital care to hospital emergency care and, ultimately, retired as an occupational healthcare administrator.

Mary is a behaviorist, having earned her Master's in Neuro-Linguistic Programming (NLP) as a board-certified practitioner and timeline therapist. She brings effective tools and techniques to our trauma-informed work, much of which she has personally developed and continues to teach and mentor within the public safety and military communities. A truly amazing healer, Mary is also a devoted wife, mother, and keeper of a small farm in the foothills of western North Carolina.

$\approx$

## Connect with Mary
*Creator and co-founder of Operation Angel Wing (OPAW)*

*Email: operationangelwing@gmail.com*
*Website: https://www.operationangelwing.org/*

$\approx$

# Your Turn

What came up for you in this story?

# CHAPTER 10
## CHOICES

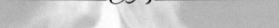

*By Justin Wood*

"The choices you make dictate the life you lead." My dad said this to me for as long as I can remember, but I would have never guessed the impact it would have on my life as I grew into the man I am today. Each day we are presented with choices, some are major, but most are trivial. Some people, like me, have had to choose whether or not living another day was an option. When I think about the road that led me to the moment I made that choice, I ask myself how I got there. It wasn't until later in my journey that I finally realized what the answer was.

Growing up, I was an athlete, participating in sports year-round—basketball, football, and baseball. My dad was my football coach; it was his niche. He was a college athlete as well as an NFL kicker. I didn't know what sport it would be; I only knew that I wanted to follow in his footsteps and make him proud. My senior year in high school, I stood on the podium at the wrestling state championships with a scholarship to Minnesota State University—Mankato. I had never felt more accomplished or prouder of my achievements. I had no idea what I was going to study in college. I only knew I had accomplished my goal.

When I arrived at school, I struggled to fit in and was having difficulties keeping up with the team. I started skipping practice, drinking, using drugs, and stopped going to class. I got my girlfriend pregnant. I was nineteen when I watched my dream slip away. I was released from the team and failed out of school, and when I got home, my problems only worsened. I started partying rather than focusing on being a dad. I would go out almost every night and drink until I couldn't feel anything. I was numbing myself from the shame I felt for failing out of school, losing my scholarship, and being nineteen with a kid. Then one day, my neighbor asked if I had ever thought about being a firefighter.

The following week I went to his station for a ride-along, and it changed the course of my life. I found something that motivated me. It wasn't the lights and sirens or the excitement of running into burning buildings. It was the feeling of being the person people called when they needed help. I felt like I had thrown my life away and was looked down upon because of it. This new path provided a way forward for me; it gave me purpose. I started the fire academy and graduated at the top of my class. Shortly after I completed EMT school, I began applying to fire departments all over Florida. While I tested and waited to be hired, I fell back into bad habits, which led to my girlfriend moving back to Minnesota with our daughter not long after I was hired.

I moved and was living alone, feeling like I did when I started college. Some nights, thoughts of worthlessness and shame crept in, and the only way I could stop those thoughts was to go out. This often led to drinking and poor decisions. I started seeing a woman who became my wife and the mother of my youngest daughter. For a few years, things began to settle down. However, when I finished paramedic school, I started to struggle again. I was having trouble letting go of certain calls and feeling, as if I had somehow failed when the call went wrong. One month, I had several pediatric calls where several ended in tragedy. I became angry and took it out on everyone around me, including my wife and kids. I was soon given leave from work to see a therapist, and I was diagnosed with PTSD, but that is about the extent of it. The therapist had a hard time understanding the First Responder culture and the amount of trauma firefighters are exposed to.

I returned to work after a few shifts, feeling like the world was watching me and no one could count on me because they thought I couldn't handle the job. I became disgruntled, angry, and unempathetic. Each time I tried to change, something would cause me to have an outburst and people would say, "See! You can't change."

So, I embraced it, thinking it was just who I was. This attitude and behavior leaked into my personal life, which led to a divorce. I felt like a failure, and I was alone again! I hurt yet another person and as a father, I now had two kids that I had failed. I went back to drinking and making poor decisions. My next relationship started out great, but it quickly deteriorated. I started to crumble, as I watched the world around me burn. I failed as a son. I failed as a husband. I failed as a father, and I had burned every bridge.

One day at work, already on thin ice, I got into an altercation with a lieutenant. The next shift I was told to go to the chief's office. When I walked through the door, both the chief and the lieutenant were waiting. My chief told me that he was ready to fire me but wanted to give me a chance to explain myself. After ten minutes, I finally broke and told him I wasn't okay, and my life was falling apart. The chief put me on leave and into our

Employee Assistance Program (EAP). I was placed with a new therapist who was better equipped for First Responders as well as a counselor. After a couple of weeks, they cleared me to return to work, but I was expected to continue seeing both. Work got better, but my personal life was suffering. My relationship with my fiancé was volatile. Eventually the two worlds—personal and professional—began to spill over.

One morning after getting off shift, I was home alone with an empty bottle of liquor, sitting on the edge of my bed with a gun in my hand. I closed my eyes and placed the gun in my mouth. I pulled the trigger and heard the "click," but nothing happened. My heart began to race, then again "click," and then a third time, "click." I opened my eyes and began to cry. I heard someone say, "They need you."

I looked down at the gun and saw the next chamber; it held my life in it. I felt numb all over, unsure of what to do next. I knew that something needed to change. So, I put the gun away and called a friend. For the first time I was honest about where I was and how I was feeling. After so many years of being in that dark place, however, I no longer knew the how or the why. My friend told me about a program in Ohio that could help. I felt a sense of relief because there was a path forward, and I chose to take it.

I was nervous to go and almost didn't get on the plane, but boarding that plane was one of the best decisions of my life. This program was an intensive, weeklong experience that I initially didn't think would work. We did a variety of activities and workshops, but there was a moment when it clicked. We did a ropes course, and part of it was climbing to the top of a telephone pole and taking a "leap of faith." As I stood at the top of that pole with my eyes closed and arms stretched out, I asked, "Why can't I let go? Why can't I change? Why can't I get my life together?" Again, I heard a voice in my head say, "You can!"

After this, I kept hearing my dad's voice over and over: "The choices we make dictate the lives we lead." On the final day of the program, we opened letters from our families, and in the stack was a letter from my dad—my mentor, my hero, and my best friend. He wrote, "The choices we make dictate the lives we lead." And it hit me.

I suddenly had the answer to why my life went the way it did and how it happened. It was me. It was the choices I made at critical moments throughout my life. For so long, I believed things happened because of the actions of others, but instead it was how I chose how to react. While this should have destroyed me, knowing I was the cause of my own self-destruction, it empowered me. I can't change what happened, but I can change where my life is going. This understanding led me to where I am today. I am now close with both my daughters and am married to an amazing woman who brought two sons into my life. The advice my dad gave me about choices when I was a child not only saved my life but changed it forever.

My dad passed shortly after I wrote this, but he was able to read it. He often spoke about his legacy and how he hoped to touch the lives of many and change the lives of some, but his biggest legacy was his children. I hope by sharing his words with others, my dad's wisdom and legacy will continue to positively impact the world.

# MEET JUSTIN WOOD

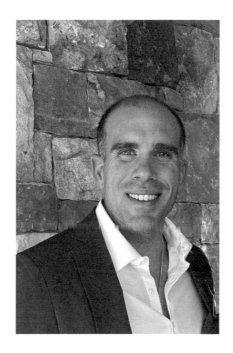

Justin Wood, a former collegiate wrestler, spent 15 years serving his community as a firefighter/paramedic in both Florida and Georgia. This profession has led Justin to become a PEER support counselor for Next Rung, allowing him to help those struggling with the same issues he struggled with for many years. His passion for helping others brought him to 62Romeo, where he facilitates an innovative sleep program that helps Veterans and First Responders build a foundation for better mental health and, ultimately, better lives. None of this would be possible without his incredible wife and four amazing children, who give him purpose every day. Justin's mantra: "Every day is a great day!"

∾

**Connect with Justin**
*Firefighter Paramedic, PEER Support Counselor*

*Email: Justin@62romeo.org*

∾

# Your Turn

What came up for you in this story?

_____
_____
_____
_____
_____
_____
_____
_____
_____
_____
_____
_____
_____
_____
_____
_____
_____
_____
_____
_____
_____
_____
_____
_____
_____

# CHAPTER 11
# FROM DARKNESS, A CALLING

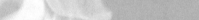

*By Todd Stewart*

"We rejoice in our sufferings knowing that suffering produces endurance, and endurance produces character, and character produces hope, and hope does not put us to shame, because God's love has been poured into our hearts through the Holy Spirit who has been given to us."

—Romans 5: 3-5*

Standing here in the light, I am grateful to God for the suffering I endured. I am grateful because I know that my suffering had purpose; I am grateful because those years spent in darkness led to a calling from God to serve my brothers and sisters.

---

\* Romans 5:3-5, English Standard Version (ESV)

Looking back, it was really a perfect setup. I am the son and grandson of sheriff's deputies in King County, Washington, a young boy who idolized his father, his hero. Becoming a First Responder was in my DNA; it was what Stewarts do. All I ever wanted was to fulfill the Stewart legacy, to serve my community, save lives, and become a hero like my father. In 1981, at seventeen years old, I became I firefighter with the Federal Way Fire Department. Six years of service resulted in thirty years of suffering. Knowing what I know now, it was suffering I would surely endure again, given God's calling on my life.

"Suck it up, rookie! The next call is coming, and it's gonna be more fucked up than the last." That was my first Critical Incident Stress Debriefing (CISD), following the suicide of a fifteen-year-old boy. I can still see his mother's face as she begged me to save him.

*Suck it up; I did.*

I was living in Station Four as a part-time firefighter. Responding 24/7 for three years was equivalent to six years as a career firefighter. SIDS, suicides, shootings, fatality DUIs—the death piled up. The lives I saved forgotten, but those I couldn't revisited me at night, pronouncing my failure. The cries of their loved ones echoed in my head. I loved my job more than anything, but I knew something wasn't right. Still, I kept my mouth shut.

*Suck it up.*

In 1985, we rolled out on yet another DUI collision. Another drunk asshole collided head-on with a young family on Interstate 5. Mom and Dad were dead, but the beautiful, young girl in the back seat was still alive. We gave it our all, but by the time we cut the roof off of the car, she had joined her parents in eternal rest.

*I snapped.*

My lieutenant pulled me off the drunk driver. He let it slide. I kept my mouth shut, but inside I screamed.

*Suck it up.*

In an instant, it was all gone—a house fire. It was an adrenaline-fueled break from the day-to-day carnage. I ran the second nozzle up the stairs in a heavily involved split level, when the stairs collapsed. I hung by my armpits and SCBA tank, my back fractured, and my legs burning up. My brothers saved my life, but there were days that followed when I wished they had let me burn.

*I was lost.*

My entire identity was being a firefighter, and it was all gone. I had "failed" to fulfill the family legacy, just as I had "failed" those I couldn't save. The nightmares became more frequent, only bloodier and soaked in death. Still, I said nothing.

*Suck it up.*

For years it went on and no one knew, not my beautiful wife, not my parents.

*No one.*

Life devolved into a meth-fueled fight to keep from sleeping. You can imagine how that worked out—divorced, estranged from my children, friends and family. In 2003, I decided to end my suffering with a .45 hollow point. That night, laying on the floor of a drug-house, God intervened. A vision of my four beautiful daughters kept that hammer from falling. And so, I decided to live and suffer. For seventeen years, I existed in a fog of nightmares and pot smoke. Waiting.

*2020 CHANGED EVERYTHING.*

Cities burned; rampant lawlessness and the pandemic (force multipliers) made an already insane world bat-shit crazy. Law enforcement officers were suddenly the enemy. Brothers and sisters were dying nearly every day, more by their own hand than by anyone else's. It wasn't any better for my beloved firefighter and EMS family. Even decades out of the fire service, every death had a profound emotional impact on me. My nightmares became more frequent, and I could not see a way out of the pain, except for ending my own life.

*It was time.*

My daughters were grown. I could finally be done with it. Was God punishing me for my failures or had He simply forgotten me? It didn't matter. Nobody would care, and I didn't blame them. I decided to free myself from the pain.

Again, God intervened. I was sitting in my truck, the pistol on my hip. It seemed to weigh one-hundred pounds. My phone rang, and I felt compelled to answer. It was my best friend, Brian, a former corrections officer.

"Hey, Brian! What's up?"

"I'm worried about you, brother," he said. "I'm seeing stuff from you that really scares me, and I just wanted to check on you and see how you're doing."

"I'm fine," I replied.

"We both know that's bullshit, brother. I love you. Tell me what's going on."

It was a buddy check, a simple gesture from someone who genuinely cared.

*Wait, someone cared?*

God was urging me to tell Brian my story, and suddenly it all came flooding out. Thirty years' worth of living in total blackness poured out, things I had never told another soul. As I spilled my "failures," shame, and self-hatred, the impenetrable darkness was pierced by the tiniest ray of light. I promised Brian I would reach out for help immediately. I was skeptical about calling my company's Employee Assistance Program. The memories that haunted me were gruesome, bloody, and filled with death. Could I inflict that on another person, even if it was their job? The EAP felt like a crap shoot. Could anyone understand what I was going through?

I called anyway.

*God was at work.*

I showed up at Peter's office convinced this was doomed to fail. Who was this guy and why did he think he could be of any help to me? I was only half listening as Peter told me about himself.

*Wait, what?*

Did he just say he was a former cop? He would understand! For the first time in a long time, I thanked God. Only He could have pulled this off.

After three weeks working with Peter, I was referred to a psychologist for diagnosis—PTSD and hyper-vigilance. Peter then introduced me to Jill, a talented trauma therapist, and we began the journey of healing my brain using EMDR. I was still living in a very dark place, but now that tiny ray of light had gotten a little brighter. A word crept into my thoughts that had not been there for thirty years—HOPE! It wasn't long until the light started to win.

*Hope is a powerful healer!*

The traumatic experiences quickly transformed from nightmare-inducing to bad but distant memories. During this time, I found my tribe—The Power of Our Story. This close-knit group of protectors welcomed me and gave me a safe space to tell my story, without shame or embarrassment. It led to amazing things.

In February of 2021, I told my story to Matt, a chaplain with the New York State Chaplain Task Force. He said, "God has a purpose for you. Use your suffering to help your First Responder family."

*I was floored!*

What happened next is hard to articulate. God's Holy Spirit

spoke to me, "Matt is speaking God's calling for you. This is the purpose the Father has prepared you for."

*I was dumbstruck.*

My years of suffering were not God's punishment, nor had He forgotten about me. My suffering had a purpose. Everything I had been through was led by God. He was equipping me for His calling. I broke down, crying.

Since that moment, God has continued to bless me. He has provided me with so many opportunities to minister, not just to First Responders but others who have lost hope, suffered from trauma, and needed a caring presence.

*God is always in charge!*

God is sovereign over all things. Your suffering has purpose! You don't know what His plan is for you, but it is a perfect plan! In His time, He will reveal His purpose for your affliction. Trust in Him.

I stand in the light of God's enduring love, the light of recovery from my suffering and the light of serving others. Were all those years of suffering worth it?

*Absolutely!*

If I had not experienced that darkness, I could not serve my brother and sister First Responders. If you are reading this, and you are suffering, know that God is with you. He has a plan for you. There is purpose in what you are going through. Let go of the shame and grasp hold of hope.

# MEET TODD STEWART

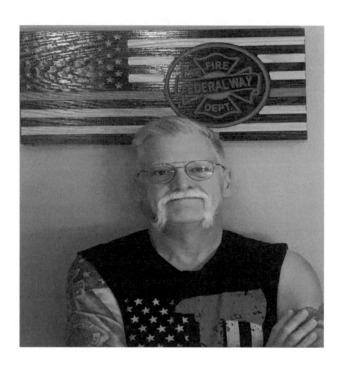

*"Free from all men, servant unto all" (1 Cor 9:19)*

Chaplain Todd "Chappie" Stewart, a Trauma Resiliency Peer Coach with 22ZERO, was born and raised in the state of Washington. He served with the Federal Way Fire Department (WA) from 1981 to 1987 and was a third generation First Responder in his family. Chappie's firefighting career was cut short by a severe back injury sustained while battling a house fire. After suffering the effects of Post-Traumatic Stress Injury (PTSI) in silence for three decades, he was finally able to get the help he needed in 2020. He lives in Waukee, Iowa and has since dedicated himself to serving his First Responder family as a chaplain with the United States Chaplain Taskforce and the First Responder's Bridge.

∿

## Connect with Todd
### Firefighter (Ret.), Chaplain

*Email: chaplainstewart@nym.hush.com*
*LinkedIn: Chaplain Todd (Chappie) Stewart CCC*

∿

# Your Turn

What came up for you in this story?

_____
_____
_____
_____
_____
_____
_____
_____
_____
_____
_____
_____
_____
_____
_____
_____
_____
_____
_____
_____
_____
_____
_____
_____

# CHAPTER 12
# CHOOSING LOVE OVER FEAR

*By*
*Holly Higgins*

"This is so hard because I love you so much, and I'm afraid."

I spoke those words on my knees in the dirt on a hot August afternoon in 2006.

Three months earlier, my eighteen-year-old son, Danny, had come home from his first year of college. New friends, new adventures, and he knew exactly what he wanted to major in. Nonetheless, he announced that he was going to "set it all aside for a few years," to enlist in the United States Air Force."

*My heart fell.*

I was the youngest child of a WWII combat Veteran who came home from war, like so many from his generation, saying nothing about the sights, sounds, smells, horrors, and atrocities that he was exposed to and sometimes participated in.

*Nothing.*
*He dealt with it.*
*He drank.*

By the time I was born, long after that war had ended, my father had become a raging, violent, and dangerous man. He eventually sought treatment but not until his addiction cost him everything, including his health. He only lived two years in sobriety. In that time, he discovered the healing power of storytelling through Alcoholics Anonymous. Shortly before he died, he told me a combat story. It answered all the whys I cried myself to sleep as a child. At twenty-one years old, I decided the US military was responsible for all the pain and damage my family suffered. After my father's flag was folded at his graveside service, I vowed never to have a relationship with that organization again.

As my bright, beautiful, son, (with the world at his feet) told me his plans to enlist, all I heard was his choice to follow in my father's footsteps. That summer, Danny discussed while I cried (and prayed) that I would find the words to talk him out of it. By summer's end, I still had not found the words.

On a hot August afternoon in 2006, while gardening, Danny quietly came out and kneeled in the dirt beside me. He put his hands in that dirt with mine and silently began pulling weeds. Being a mom, I knew what that meant. He wanted something. I knew what he wanted. He wanted confirmation that I would come to his swearing-in ceremony. He was part of a group of exceptional recruits invited to be sworn in by a General at a special ceremony in front of dignitaries at the Chicago Air and Water Show. He wanted me there. While we continued to pull weeds silently, he waited, and I looked up at that deep, blue sky, and pleaded for the "magic words" that would change his mind.

"This is so hard," I said. "Because I love you so much, and I am afraid." The moment I spoke those words, I remembered what I'd taught Danny about love and fear. Those words did not change his mind; they changed my heart. Because my love for him is so much greater than fear, I told my son I would be at that ceremony.

The following weekend, my husband and I stood on a hot, sandy beach in Chicago, and watched what was, at that time, the most honorable and noble ceremony we had ever witnessed. Afterwards, I told Danny that I was humbled.

Several months later, we were at Lackland Air Force Base where Danny graduated from basic training in the top ten percent! He stood so straight and tall in his crisp, new uniform and talked to me about what integrity meant to him. His transformation was impressive, and I told him so.

Months later, we were at the Naval School Explosive Ordnance Disposal, also known in the military as EOD— Bomb Squad to us civilians. EOD is one of the most difficult technical schools in the Department of Defense. Historically, the EOD technical training program has a seventy-five percent attrition rate, meaning for every five hundred Airmen enrolled in the program, one hundred and twenty-five finish. Fifty-one percent fail the first phase. Danny sailed through and graduated with honors. I told him how proud I was to be his mom.

When Danny deployed, he knew I was concerned about how combat would affect his heart, mind, and spirit. So, before each deployment, he'd say, "Remember, mom; I'm going to save lives, not take them."

On October 5, 2010, while deployed to Afghanistan, after a long day of disarming IEDs (Improvised Explosive Device), the team was ready to call it. They had disarmed six IEDs that day. The military estimates an average of five lives saved per IED safely disarmed. The bomb dog appeared confused earlier and continued to return to a specific area, indicating a threat. The equipment wasn't picking anything up. The combat engineer checked several times and found nothing. So, they called it a day.

Danny's EOD team was attached to the Canadian Army for that mission, and he had befriended several of the Canadian soldiers. One of those soldiers made plans with Danny to meet his brothers in northern Minnesota after the war. The Canadians were leaving the next day, so Danny told his teammates that he was going over to say goodbye. As he walked toward the Canadians, Danny passed the area where the dog had indicated something unusual.

That's when my son stepped on the pressure plate.

There was only one life lost in that blast.

I spent many months in a fog, remembering very little. In fact, I have only three clear memories from that time. My first memory was when the military told me that Danny's face was untouched, and though his body was so badly injured it could not sustain his life, he was lucid enough to draw on his EMT training from college and instruct his teammates on how to save his life. I had a hard time believing the military. I was haunted by the fact that Danny's casket was closed. I never got to see that beautiful face again. If what they told me was true, then why the closed casket? After my father's experience, how could I trust them?

My second memory was walking out of the chapel at Vandenberg Air Force Base following Danny's military funeral. His Commanding Officer's wife approached me with a message from the medivacs. They wanted Danny's mom to know that as they loaded him onto the transport, they told him, "You're going home, son." He replied, "I know, but please tell my mom that I didn't break my face". Danny took his last breath minutes later. That message caused an about-face in my journey with the US Military. Danny's message couldn't possibly have been made up. It was a family joke that started the summer he turned five. We lived on top of a hill that his older brothers would race down on their two-wheel bikes. The day we took the training wheels off Danny's bike, I told him, "You aren't ready for that hill. Stay here with me and your little brother until your balance is better."

In the split second it took me to look back at his little brother riding in circles on his tricycle, Danny darted down that hill, racing out of control with the front wheel wobbling the whole way down. He wiped out in the gravel at the bottom. I sprinted after him and held him in my lap while he cried. Half his face was covered in road rash, and when he fought to catch his breath, he cried, "Pfpfpfpfpf... I'm not even five yet, and I aweady bwoke my face." From that day on, before every trip away from home (including deployments), I'd always tell him, "Don't break your face."

The message from the medivacs was powerful. The military did not lie. Danny knew he was dying, and he sent me a message that only he could send. He truly was calm, just as they had reported. And he was peaceful, even to the end; so much so that he never even lost his sense of humor.

My third memory is when the fog lifted, and I was able to articulate the words, "I am grateful I supported my son on his journey with the United States Military." Those words baffled some. Someone said, "If he hadn't been in the military, he wouldn't have been in Afghanistan and died at twenty-three years old."

Perhaps. However, I am (and will forever be) grateful that on that hot August afternoon in 2006, I chose love over fear. Had I not, Danny still would have gone to that swearing-in ceremony. But I would have missed it. He still would have graduated from basic training in the top ten percent and stood straight and tall in his crisp, new uniform and talked about what integrity meant to him. He just wouldn't have been able to talk to me about it. And I wouldn't have a precious memory from the end of that weekend, when, after we hugged goodbye, he glided away and my husband leaned down and whispered in my ear, "He left home a boy; look at that confident man." Danny still would have graduated with honors from the EOD school. I would have missed that awe-inspiring ceremony. And he still would have been deployed to Afghanistan and been killed in action on that dusty road 7,000 miles from home. The only difference is that he would have died having never heard me tell him how proud I was of the man he had become.

I am forever grateful I chose love over fear. I've accepted the lessons grief has taught me; I've discovered that love is not only greater than fear, but it is also greater than death. Through love, gratitude, and telling Danny's story, I have a restored sense of hope, meaning and purpose which enables me to enjoy all that remains. All this because of my son and my hero—Senior Airman Daniel J. Johnson.

# MEET HOLLY HIGGINS

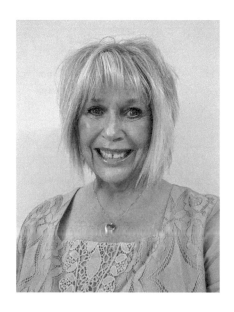

Holly Higgins is a Gold Star mom, keynote speaker, program manager and lead story coach for The Heroes Journey Storytelling Workshops, and liaison for Families of the Fallen with Pineapple Express Relief. Holly serves veterans, first responders, and families of our nation's fallen by "unlocking the timeless healing power of storytelling." Holly worked for over 25 years as a registered nurse and social worker in the mental health field. While serving others, she has found healing in her own journey.

Holly's son, Senior Airman Daniel J. Johnson, was killed in

action in Afghanistan, and it was his tragic, untimely death that taught her that grief is not something to avoid but rather embrace. In embracing her own pain, she learned that grief is a gift. She believes it helps us to mourn our loved ones. It teaches and guides us as we navigate loss, sadness, and unspeakable tragedy. Daniel's courage, patriotism, and integrity inspire Holly every day to live a life that is worthy of his sacrifice. He is her hero because he loved his country enough to die for it.

∾

### *Connect with Holly*
**Gold Star Mom of SrA Daniel J Johnson**

**Story Coach and Public Speaker**

*Email: hollyhiggins@live.com*
*LinkedIn: Holly Higgins-Staudacher*
*Facebook: Holly Mae Staudacher*

∾

# Your Turn

What came up for you in this story?

_____

_____

_____

_____

_____

_____

_____

_____

_____

_____

_____

_____

_____

_____

_____

_____

_____

_____

_____

_____

_____

_____

_____

_____

# CHAPTER 13

# CARRYING HIS LEGACY: A SISTER'S JOURNEY THROUGH LOSS AND HEALING

*By*

*Melissa Ketchel*

On the evening of November 17, 2004, I put my fifteen-month-old son to bed, read my daughter *Bear Wants More*, and prayed for the safety of her uncle Michael, my younger brother who was deployed for the second time to Iraq, this time participating in the Second Battle of Fallujah. I then fell asleep beside her. My youngest brother was sleeping on the couch. I woke up not long after to the sound of my house phone ringing—continually. And then my cell phone was ringing, one after the other, making it impossible to sleep. The cell service at my small rental house was not very good. I could see I had a voicemail but had to leave the house to check it. Driving down the dirt road, I thought I would ride around the block and check my messages. The first message was from a buddy, checking to see what I was up to on the weekend. The next message was my ex-husband. The message was cryptic, his voice softer than normal.

"I heard something about your brother, and I am not sure if it's true; just call me back."

I quickly dialed his number, and he answered with the same soft voice, despite me yelling, "What did you hear?"

He stuttered, " I am not sure if it is true or not …"

His voice faded off.

I screamed into the receiver as I made a left turn for the second time.

"Just tell me!"

Stoically, he replied, "Melissa, your brother is dead."

*No … not my brother.*

I heard the words but couldn't quantify them. Not Michael! Not my best friend, my partner in crime, the keeper of my past and all my secrets. How could he be gone from this world? How could he leave me? A lifetime of memories with him flashed before my eyes—hiding under the Christmas tree, trying to catch Santa Claus, wiffle ball on the neighbor's lawn that their dad mowed into a baseball field. Running wild in the neighborhood until the streetlights came on. The time when, as teenagers, we almost burned down a forest and laughed together after my mom spanked us with a plastic spatula, both of us fake crying because it didn't hurt. The last time I saw him, he was standing on the side of the road. We were leaving a bar; he was going to my parents' house, and I was going home. Michael pulled over to give me a CD. He had another copy in California, so he was giving it to me. I have never been a hugger, but when he got out of the car, I hugged him. We laughed and drove our separate ways, saying the words "See you later."

*Later would never come.*

There is a distinct "before and after" and a sea of "what ifs." What if he didn't go back? What if he didn't play the hero that day? What if he didn't reenlist to stay with his men? What if he just came home?

Simple tasks, such as getting out of bed and getting dressed became monumental challenges. The world carries on, people go to work, laugh, make dinner and smile. While in grief, I was suspended in a state of disbelief. Each day, I woke up and before my eyes would open, it would hit me again.

*My brother was dead.*

The grief washed over me until I was numb. Losing Michael shattered our family in ways we couldn't have imagined. My younger brother turned to drugs. My parents divorced, and my plans for the future felt like they evaporated overnight. I thought I might die myself from sadness, a pain worse than any physical pain I had ever experienced. My kids were the reason I got out of bed in the morning, but I was only going through the motions, not truly living.

Then one day, I heard Michael's words looping in my mind, "Everyone needs someone to confess to." He spoke those words to me two years earlier. October 8, 2002, on Failaka Island near Kuwait, US Marines were part of a training exercise. One of these Marines was my brother—Michael Hanks. He joined the Marine Corps in January of the previous year before the horrors of 9/11. During a lull in their training, the Marines were playing a game of stickball when two Kuwaiti men opened fire on them. Two Marines were shot, and one Marine, Tony Sledd, was fatally wounded. Although the war in Iraq had not officially begun, Sledd's killing has been remembered by some as the first American casualty of the Second Iraq War. That day was a baptism by fire into war for those Marines. Sledd became a rallying cry as the 3rd Battalion 1st Marines went into Baghdad the following year.

Between this training and being deployed into the initial invasion of Iraq, Michael came home to Michigan for a brief leave. While home, he came to my house for dinner. I was pregnant with my second child and fully emerged into my life as a wife and mother. During this visit, Michael told me he needed to talk and looked at me in such a way that I knew it was going to be something I didn't want to hear. I didn't want to hear about war, or insurgents, or people dying. I wanted to live in the blissful reality of my own ignorance. In a moment that I will never forget, he stopped and grabbed my arm. His six foot one inch frame was much taller than mine at five foot seven inches. He looked downward, into my eyes with desperation. He said, "Everyone needs someone to confess to." For him, it was me. Feeling the seriousness of the moment, we went for a drive to talk because its private in a car, and you don't have to look into the eyes of the person you are talking to. As I suspected, he told me about war, what happened on that fateful day on Failaka Island, how people he loved died, and how his brothers captured and killed the insurgents that attacked them. That conversation would change the trajectory of my life. I just didn't know it yet.

One day, in the aftermath of his death, I decided to become the person for whom to confess, for all those who served with Michael. I just started showing up, inviting myself to California. Going to Vegas with several of those he served with. Forging friendships over the phone with these men, my brother's brothers. I often joked that I was the sister they never wanted but were stuck with. I quickly learned that my relationship with these men was just as meaningful for them as it was for me. We helped each other heal.

The pain and heartbreak of losing my brother to war has been profound. It is not just him that I've lost but the entire future I once envisioned, where our children would grow up together. He loved his role as Uncle, showering my kids with love and affection. I will never forget him, this big, tough Marine, flying from California to Michigan with a massive teddy bear on his lap—a Christmas gift for my daughter. When my parents and younger brother drive me crazy, I get angry at Michael for leaving me. But at the same time, he gave me this incredible gift of friendship in those who served alongside him.

We laugh, cry, and call each other during the good times and the bad. I get to watch their children grow up and get the honorary title of Aunt Melissa. Some of these children's first or middle names are Michael. My children have grown up in the safety and protection of knowing that these Marines will show up to protect them. My daughter, Makiah, now twenty-two, was four when Michael died. She would often tell people that she had "nineteen uncles and seventeen of them are Marines."

I live a privileged life that was paid for first by my brother's blood ... and then by my actions of showing up and holding space for the men who would trade places with Michael if given the choice. Together, we're carrying on Michael's legacy, honoring his memory and continuing to build the bond we've forged in loss, a bond strengthened by love and shared commitment. Nearly twenty years later, not a week goes by that I don't speak to one of the guys who served with Mike.

Many combat Veterans struggle with survivors' guilt, haunted by both the memories of war and those that they fought alongside who never made it home. This guilt often prevents them from reaching out to the families of the fallen. These families, like mine, who have lost their loved ones in service, share a profound understanding of sacrifice, honor, and the enduring impact of war. I would encourage any Veteran to reach out to Gold Star Families. By reaching out, you honor the sacrifice of their loved one and help them (and yourself) heal. I was often told, "But I don't want to remind you of your brother's death." Hearing from those he served with does not remind me that my brother is dead. It reminds me that he lived.

# MEET MELISSA HANKS KETCHEL

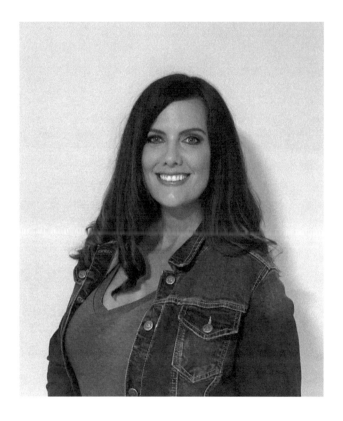

Melissa Hanks Ketchel is a Gold Star sister, devoted Veteran advocate and keynote speaker who lost her brother, Lance Corporal Michael W. Hanks, in Fallujah, Iraq in 2004. Melissa specializes in non-traditional mental healthcare. She is certified in Neuro-Linguistic Programming (NLP) and trained in mental health first aid and suicide intervention, As a Veteran community program director for a mortgage company, she excels in VA home loans.

Melissa serves as the vice president of the 3rd Battalion 1st Marines Association and is the founder of the Michael Wayne Hanks Legacy Foundation. Her deep involvement with Gold Star Families and Veteran organizations helps to keep the memory of her brother close. She is honored and always open to sharing her story of restoring meaning and purpose after a profound loss. Melissa lives in Huntington Beach, California.

∼

### *Connect with Melissa*
*Veteran Advocate - Gold Star Sister of LCPL Michael W. Hanks*

*Email: melketchel@gmail.com*
*LinkedIn: https://linktr.ee/melketchel*

∼

# Your Turn

What came up for you in this story?

# CHAPTER 14
## OUR SECOND CHANCES

*By*

*Scott Duncan*

A significant emotional event at the age of eleven put me on the path to not becoming a victim of loss in this life. I recall the moment well, as I woke up at around 2 a.m. to the sound of my parents arguing. I'd never heard this before. Evidently, they argued as a couple, but their quarrels never happened around my older brother and me—this was different. As I opened my bedroom door and peeked down the hall into the den, I saw my mom crying while she was ironing my father's Air Force uniform. As my mom verbally pushed back against my dad, which she never did in public, he slapped her on the face. I couldn't believe my eyes. My heart exploded in my chest. I will not go any further into the painful specifics of what happened moments later, except to say it was truly an out of body experience for me and certainly for my mom.

After receiving a call, my dad went into my parents' bedroom to pack his suitcase. At that moment, I mustered up the courage to confront him, which my brother and I never did. I walked into the room and found him feverishly packing his clothing. I asked him what he was doing—why was he packing? He chose to lie and tell me he had to go on TDY (official military travel). He didn't realize I had seen his actions and listened to the words between him and my mom. He also didn't have the courage to tell me the truth. I called him a liar; he noticed my right hand clinched tightly into a fist. He said, "So, you want to hit me, huh?"

As I wiped away my tears, I replied, "I want to knock the s#!t out of you, but I know what will happen if I try!" My words and anger caught my dad off guard, and it stopped him in his tracks. I realized I had willfully crossed the line and took the opportunity to quickly retreat to my room, praying that he would not follow me.

A few minutes later I heard his footsteps drumming down the hall. Thankfully, he went past my room and out the front door—gone forever—in so many ways. He died seven years later, at the age of forty-two. I was a senior in high school. I found out my dad passed away on the evening of my maternal grandfather's birthday—who was a Marine. We were celebrating and had just cut the birthday cake—strawberry shortcake, Granddaddy's favorite!

As the cake was being served, the phone rang. I jumped up to answer it, thinking it was my buddy, Bob. We had plans to head out later that evening; the following day was "Senior Skip Day." I had been looking forward to this much-needed distraction. The call was from my dad's friend at church. The gentleman was very direct and to the point, informing me my dad had just passed away. An awkward silence followed. I thanked him for the call and hastily hung up.

I knew my dad had been diagnosed with stage-four lung cancer. In fact, he called my brother and me five months earlier, during the Christmas holiday, to inform us that he was terminally ill and had about five months left to live. My brother was in the Army at the time and was home on leave. This revelation made that Christmas feel somber, and I was glad my brother was home with me and Mom.

Hanging up the phone, I proceeded to my bedroom and lost it. It was a brief and painfully quiet cry, as I didn't want to draw attention to the bad news and ruin my wonderful grandfather's birthday celebration. As things would have it, this was also the evening prior to Senior Prom.

*Ugh!*

So, I put on the false face I had crafted over the years to mask my pain. This mask was a result of many notions: the need for a self-defense mechanism; the necessity to hide my humiliation of not having a father; and the fact that I felt the obligation to be strong for my mom all of those years in between.

I had spent seven years without a dad. During that time, we had been on government assistance. My mom, a housewife for seventeen years, was pushed into the workforce with minimal skills. She suffered greatly in the years that followed because she truly loved my dad. But she became strong and did not leave my brother and me. She was not a quitter. She loved us.

In those tough and formative years, I learned the value of hard work. I was a fifth grader, picking up a paper route and cutting other people's lawns in the neighborhood. Over the summers, while working for my grandfather, I painted houses. I always had a job. I learned to clean the house, wash my own clothes, and maintain the yard and car. I learned responsibility and self-reliance. I also spent many days and nights alone. That was a difficult cross to bear, and it was lonely.

The silver lining in all that took place was that my dad found

God through the forgiveness of Jesus in the last two to three years of his life. He was truly a changed man, and that would bring me peace on many levels. I discovered that Dad did love me and that he was sorry for what he had put us all through. He asked for forgiveness. This lifted a yoke off of my shoulders, a heavy one steeped in hatred. A burden that would have steered my life to a very bad outcome.

Although many difficulties came as a result of growing up without a dad, I was blessed to have a mom, a brother, and grandparents who loved me. I also had best friends, especially Mark and Bob. By the grace of God, we are still best of friends today. Furthermore, there were key men in my life who helped shape my character, men like my grandfather, the minister of music at our church (Don Laine), my high school football and track coach (George Versprillie), and the dads of my two best friends, Cliff and Bob, Sr. These men were role models for me as a young man. To this day, I remain amazed at the wisdom they imparted to me.

Life moved forward, and I would go on to college, get married, become a Marine officer, and my wife and I would eventually have two incredible daughters. In my twenty-one years of active-duty military service, I deployed around the world and served in combat operations. Through those years, there were Marines and Sailors I knew and worked with who lost their lives. Some died in combat, others died during training, and, unfortunately, too many died by suicide.

In order to keep my wits about me and remain the leader that I was required to be in those moments and over time, I learned to handle these significant events by compartmentalizing them into "buckets." Looking back, I can truly say that God has granted me a sense of serenity and acceptance in coping with loss. When I learned to trust God in all matters, it took the heavy burden off my shoulders. We live our lives with free will. Yet, we are not alone in our struggles as I once thought I was as a young boy. The grace and forgiveness I have found in Jesus has transformed my life and mindset.

I learned a remarkable lesson. Don't turn down an invitation to reconnect with a family member once there has been a rift in the relationship. Obviously, if there are questions or concerns for safety, that's quite different. I know for a fact that the forgiveness I found for my dad was laid on my heart from God. Many things had to come together for me to see my dad anew, to give him a second chance. I had sworn my dad off because he deserted me. It was actually because of my grandfather's actions that I gave my dad one more shot. He convinced me that my dad had changed. Granddaddy said it was worth my time to spend a week with him during Christmas; the following Christmas, my dad was diagnosed with cancer.

Remember, my grandfather was my mom's dad, how significant is that? He had keenly felt the pain of betrayal my mother experienced, and he saw firsthand his daughter's brokenness. How could he offer such sound and loving advice? I was upset with my grandfather for what I felt was bad advice, and I thought that he did not understand my pain. No. He understood all too well. Granddaddy was there, helping to put the pieces back together. After all, he survived the Battle of Tarawa during WWII.

That Christmas with my dad, combined with the realization years later that "God has a plan," forever changed my perspective on our second chances in life and the need for patience, grace, and forgiveness. Made simple: Reach out. Be willing. Be open. I learned to trust and love others again through my faith in God. He performs miracles.

# MEET SCOTT DUNCAN

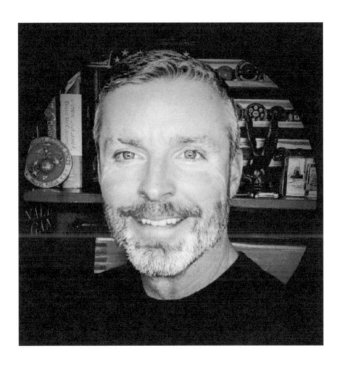

Scott Duncan, a Retired Lieutenant Colonel, served in the Marine Corps for 21 years as a logistician. He commanded at the company and battalion levels and served in combat operations in Iraq. Scott entered the "Veteran space" upon transitioning from military service in 2012. He directed and co-founded two non-profits focused on recruiting, training, and placing Veterans into the renewable energy sector, and eventually partnered with the Department of Energy in the Solar Ready Vets program.

He is a consultant to businesses and government entities on the subject of hiring Veterans, developing recruiting, training, fundraising, and placement strategies. He is a social media content creator and podcast host of *What's Next?—Beyond Service*, working alongside The Power of Our Story, interviewing prior service members, First Responders, and spouses, as well as speaking to the challenges of transition to civilian life and employment. Scott is a keynote speaker on Veteran's issues and the importance of America and its founding.

∾

### *Connect with Scott*
**LtCol USMC (Ret.)**

*LinkedIn: Scott Duncan (MPA)*

∾

# Your Turn

What came up for you in this story?

_____
_____
_____
_____
_____
_____
_____
_____
_____
_____
_____
_____
_____
_____
_____
_____
_____
_____
_____
_____
_____
_____
_____
_____
_____
_____

# CHAPTER 15
# FAITH, FORGIVENESS, AND LETTING GO

*By*

*Lona Spisso*

I have vivid memories as a child—crawling under my bed, clinging to my blanket, crying myself to sleep. I am a twin and was the youngest child of four when my parents divorced. It was terrifying when Mom left. I clung to her leg, begging her not to go when we saw her. I wore my Wonder Woman pajamas; they made me feel like a superhero. Yet inside I was just a little girl, self-soothing. Not having a mom at home was hard. Dad loved us but didn't always know the right things to say or do. My biggest insecurity was my fear of being abandoned again.

Shortly after my parent's divorced, we lost my mom's sister to suicide. Then, we lost my mom's brother, my favorite uncle, to suicide a few years later. I was ten. It was so confusing. They invented a story of his death; suicide was seen as a disgrace and embarrassment. I didn't know how to navigate shame.

*Were we really that dysfunctional family?*

This exacerbated my abandonment wounds, causing me to jump into a "fixer" role to keep me from being hurt again. My dad, a business owner, worked tirelessly—sun-up to sun-down. Us kids were raised by a stream of nannies, furthering my abandonment issues. In high school, I was forced to take on the role of "mother hen." I looked forward to dad being away for work; it meant no yelling. Dad had anger issues. The yelling, pushing, and repeated put downs slayed me. He'd say, "You're never going to amount to anything."

I moved out immediately after high school. Driven and determined, I excelled in college. However, I still struggled with unhealthy coping skills. I wanted to feel accepted. I needed a secret weapon to avoid vulnerability and rejection at all costs! I thought, *I can find this in the military.* Dad scoffed, "You'll never make it through basic training!"

In 2000, with a few college degrees under my belt, I enlisted in the US Army. I embraced the military. It challenged me and provided structure. I got into Officer's Candidate School. I was going to prove my dad wrong.

### I WAS *worthy!*

My service gave me confidence. I learned how to be compassionate, which accelerated my leadership roles. There was never a problem that couldn't be solved, and I was never nervous about saying, "No." Problem solving has always been one of my superpowers.

In 2002, I met a great classmate and fellow officer named Danny. He became a good friend. I'll tell you more about him later. Around the same time, I met my husband (now former), who will remain nameless. This man had charisma, confidence, and looks that would turn heads. His flattery left me on an emotional high and gave me the self-esteem I longed for. He was the first man I truly felt safe with; I was able to drop my armor and reveal my wounds. His words of affirmation were exactly what I needed.

Seven years later, we were married. Soon after we said, *"I do,"* his whole demeanor changed. I knew something was off but couldn't put my finger on it. He began isolating me from family and friends. While he made me think I was the center of his universe, his manipulations were cruel and deliberate. Leaving wasn't an option. My Christian values taught me to stay married. Plus, I desperately wanted to break my family cycle of divorce. So, I suppressed my feelings and went back to being a self-soother.

A year into my marriage, my husband and I were both deployed to Afghanistan. He was a Sergeant Major. He also knew Danny, who I mentioned earlier. After a hot, twelve-hour day in July, I was feeling exhausted and hungry. I ran to the chow hall, where I bumped into Danny. He was sitting alone. When I walked towards him, he looked up and smiled at me. I sat down, and it was like no time had passed since I'd seen him last. We had a great time catching up. Danny was one of the most selfless guys I knew, the kind of guy who had boot marks on his back from always being the first to carry others' struggles. A few hours later, Danny was gone.

*How could I not see one single sign that he was about to take his own life?*

I would have "carried him as far as he needed," if only I had known.

*Once again, suicide was at my doorstep.*

It was all so disorienting; it threw me into another emotional spiral. My heart was broken. I suffered intense feelings of sadness and guilt. I truly believed I could have stopped it from happening, had I seen the signs. But we all know that is most likely not the case.

As I continued to work through my grief, our deployment was over, and we were heading home. I needed my husband to be there for me. He just wanted me to move past it and focus on being his wife. He always needed to be the center of attention. He loved to draw an audience. He would snap and defend criticism from others, responding with a back-handed statement. He always told me he was misunderstood. Not knowing I was married to a covert narcissist, I believed him.

From that point forward, self-soothing and fixing others' problems provided a sense of purpose and validation. I did all of the work inside and outside of the house, while he took care of himself. I avoided conflict at all costs to reduce any chance of him abandoning me. I didn't want to be that little girl hiding under the bed again. He knew this about me. He knew exactly what to say and do to keep me tied to him. Life was a roller coaster, full of highs and lows. Then one morning, after he left for work, I walked into the bedroom from the shower to find his wedding ring on the nightstand.

*What the Fuck? He never takes his ring off*

He didn't even have the courage to speak to me or leave a note. I went into our walk-in closet and saw a gaping hole where his custom-tailored suits and shirts once hung. They were gone. I felt the blood drain from my face. I sat on the bed, paralyzed. I had been blindsided, devastated when I found out about the multiple affairs. Within days, I had zero access to our finances.

*Good Lord, how long had he been planning this?*

Fifteen years of my life gone in the blink of an eye. The next several years were some of the lowest of my life. He didn't want to let me go, yet still having the affairs and using our business and finances to keep me in bondage. As a leadership coach, I wasn't practicing what I preached to my clients. As a woman, I no longer recognized myself. I became co-dependent, filled with panic and uncertainty, completely paralyzed with fear to set boundaries.

For three-and-a-half years, he dragged me in and out of our divorce. Suddenly, I had a profound awakening. I reached radical acceptance. The man was incapable of changing, and the love he had for me was an illusion. I was allowing him to steal my joy. Scared to death, I took my first steps back into my power. I knew I had to cut off all ties. It was through the grace of God that my heart began to heal. Through years of counseling and hard work, I was finally free from his *trauma bond* and rage. I started to take better care of myself.

*Mindset is powerful!*

We stand in our power when we successfully align our minds with our values and behaviors. The pinnacle of healing started once I learned what forgiveness truly meant. Forgiveness is *not* how you feel about the abuser, justifying their actions, letting them off the hook, or even letting them back into your life. Forgiveness is about your freedom and letting go of what no longer serves you. Allowing forgiveness in my heart completely changed the course of my life.

Then, God almost immediately dropped an amazing man into my life, someone who has shown me the true meaning of loyalty, faith and action. And I've never been happier! His name is Rob. I'm no longer that little girl hiding under the bed. I have amazing relationships with both my mom and dad. Letting go and removing people and things that no longer serve you is like pruning a tree to help it grow.

Everyone's journey is different. It took me almost seven years to broach this subject without shame. I'm not a victim; I'm a victor—no regrets! These lessons made me a better woman and coach. I would not be where I am today without the hardships and pain. There is no instruction manual or timeline for grief and loss. So, always listen to your gut and **NEVER** ignore the red flags. I embrace my scars and keep moving forward. Getting to the other side of grief and forgiveness brings about absolute freedom.

# MEET LONA SPISSO

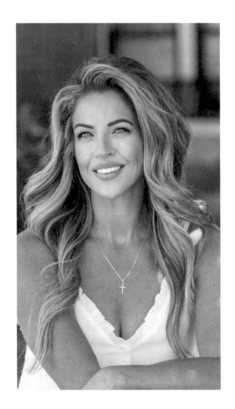

For over two decades, Lona has empowered current and rising leaders with critical action steps to achieve both personal and professional goals. She has coached in the private, corporate, military, and professional sports industries to help her clients break through plateaus and achieve extraordinary growth. She has coached individuals and teams during many phases of organizational change and challenges, such as IPOs, mergers, RIFs, sector switching, and transitioning Veterans from the military. Lona relies on her expertise in human behavior, her background in psychology, as well as her experience as a former Army officer and Combat Veteran. She develops relationships quickly, identifies obstacles and creates strategic action plans guiding her clients to success. Lona is unparalleled in her ability to provide customized solutions for leaders and teams. This approach includes aligning mindsets, behaviors, and actions with core values. When these four elements align, she believes profound leaps in leadership become possible and true personal transformation begins. Her straightforward approach with structure, accountability, compassion, and transparency, blended with proven performance strategies generates real results. Lona arms her clients with precise skills to navigate and overcome any challenge that comes their way, while helping them build the quality of life they've always dreamed of. If you would like to connect with Lona, please reach out to her through any of the following channels.

≈

### Connect with Lona
**Leadership Coach & Combat Veteran**

*Email: info@EliteLeadershipTraining.com*
*LinkedIn: Lona Spisso*
*FaceBook: Elite Leadership Training*
*InstaGram: @lonaspisso*

≈

# Your Turn

What came up for you in this story?

_____

_____

_____

_____

_____

_____

_____

_____

_____

_____

_____

_____

_____

_____

_____

_____

_____

_____

_____

_____

_____

_____

_____

_____

_____

_____

# CHAPTER 16
## SILENT BATTLE CRY

—∞—

*By*
*Lakeydra Houston*

I never thought I would sign on the dotted line to serve my country, but anything was better than being home. I was fading away—broken and tired from using drugs to numb the pain. Volleyball was my escape, but I was failing college.

*What was left for me?*

The Air Force. It was my time to break free, prove that I would not fail. How could I have known my life would change forever? On January 8, 2002, my emotions were running high.

*Was joining the military the right decision?*

While in training, I received a letter from my grandmother, telling me that she was proud of me and to keep going. That was my fuel; I couldn't let her down! After a few months, I graduated and officially became Airman Strange. Tears flowed as I watched my family walk toward me.

*I did it!*

Later that day, I was eating with my family. I noticed that my deaf, younger sister seemed distant. She was there, but her emotions were not. My mother pulled me aside and told me to sit down. I knew something was wrong; it all felt so familiar.

"Keke, your sister was raped," my mother said. "We wanted to wait until after you graduated to tell you."

*I lost it.*

Guilt ran through my body. I felt like I hadn't protected her. I ran to my little sister and hugged her. Our tears soaked into my uniform. That's when the flashbacks began. For me, leaving home meant not having to see my cousins (the perpetrators) again. I felt my sister's pain—not being believed, people turning their backs on her, and thinking it was her fault.

At the age of six, my body had reactions I wasn't ready for, and I couldn't describe the feeling. I was groomed to believe I was beautiful and my "bedroom eyes" drew my perpetrators to me. I was confused. I couldn't comprehend if what they did was good or bad since they were the only two male cousins to touch me. I was told that I would get in trouble, and they would hurt me if I said something. I knew it was wrong, but I stayed silent. The abuse went on for a few years, and my attitude changed. I became defiant until, at the age of thirteen, after watching a similar story on Oprah, I found the strength to tell my family. In the back of my mind, I knew the cops would be called, and I could finally have justice.

*No.*

Instead, the secret continued, and no one seemed to believe me. So, now my sister was hurting. I should have protected her. I felt like I had failed her. After she and I spent some time together, I reminded her that I believed her and promised to take care of her. She signed to me that she was proud of me and wanted me to keep going.

Sexual harassment seemed like the norm in military technical school. I was so naïve. When it happened to me, I thought it was just some guy showing interest, smacking me on the butt and acting out in sexually suggestive ways. I felt wanted and admired. After a few months, I was informed that I received my first duty assignment. I just knew it would be Texas!

Instead, the Airforce said, "You are going to Tucson Arizona!"

*My heart dropped.*

I wasn't ready to be away from my supportive family. In the back of my mind, I wanted to go Absent Without Leave (AWOL), but I knew I had nothing to go back to.

*Arizona ... here I come.*

As I arrived at the base, I felt like fresh meat in a meat market. It was uncomfortable. I focused on learning my job and getting settled in. A few days later, I met the leadership team and started processing. While making introductions, I felt uncomfortable with one person in particular. I went to his office to get his signature, and as he stood up from his desk, I could clearly see he was attracted to me. He walked over to where I stood and proceeded to fix the ribbons on my blues jacket, brushing the back of his hand across my breasts. I moved, thinking it may have been an accident, but he continued advancing. I ran out of his office—confused.

*Why was this happening again?*

Did I show some interest? Did I flirt without realizing it? A young, female Airman, picking up trash, saw me leaving. She told me not to say anything or I would get kicked out. As I walked to my dorm room, so many things ran through my mind. I felt silenced again, and the six-year-old me resurfaced.

On my first day of work, a few of the guys asked if I had met the leader who touched my breasts. Not knowing he had already made a move, they warned me to be careful around him because he was "nasty." I remained silent. As months passed, I started crossing the border to Mexico. I was drinking a lot to cope with the pain. I didn't care that I was underage; I wanted the pain to stop.

After a few days on leave, one of my coworkers came to me. He seemed "off." When I asked him about it, he said we'd talk after work. That never happened. Not long after I relieved him from lunch, I heard a scream over the radio. "He shot himself! He has no pulse."

*I couldn't believe it.*

I went by my coworker's post and saw the bullet hole and blood pouring from the gate shack. I was not ready for him to go. I never received the "required" therapy following that incident, so I continued to drink heavier until I had no choice but to quit. Shortly after my coworker's suicide, I found myself pregnant and in an abusive marriage. I was broken; I wasn't ready to raise a kid. I was not emotionally equipped. After having my son, I received orders to deploy to Korea to get away from my abusive husband. That military tour caused me to spiral out of control. Korea was the assignment every service member wanted. Drinking was encouraged. Leaving my son with my grandparents was my only option; I was selfish and needed to figure myself out. I was so excited to start over and learn, but a few months after arriving, a group of fellow Airmen took me out to "welcome" me to the unit, including one woman who was a friend of mine from my previous base. Knowing she was there, and she had my back, gave me the green light, so I embraced the moment.

I remember drinking and getting drunk quicker than normal. The room was spinning, but I wasn't worried because my girlfriend was there. The next morning, however, I woke up nude and in pain. I was in a guy's room—someone I didn't know. I rushed out of there and went to my girlfriend, asking her what had happened. Instead of comforting me, I was called a slut. "You asked for it," she said.

I couldn't report the rape because I was told by multiple people that I had initiated it. I was ashamed and that young child inside of me was screaming for help. I was useless as both a woman and a mother

*How could I let this continue to happen to me?*

Before my tour ended in Korea, I was raped two more times, and in those moments, I felt like I deserved it. No one would believe me if I had said anything because I was known as the "dorm party girl." As I packed up to close that chapter of my life, I was finally able to see my son, but I was absent. I did not love myself. I was emotionally detached from him. I was the parent I never wanted to be. My grandparents gave my son the love he needed.

In 2009, I was fighting for my life; I wanted to be better. A phone call from my mother was rare, but one day she called screaming and crying.

"She's dead," she said. "Your sister is dead."

I was not ready for this. I was trying to heal. After my sister's funeral, I put a gun to my head, wanting to end it all. I did not care about the pain my son, or my family would feel.

*The pain needed to end.*

As I was getting ready to pull the trigger, my ex-husband wrestled the gun away. I was angry, looking for other ways to die by suicide. I got on my knees and screamed at God. I was so angry with Him for leaving me as a child ... and during multiple sexual assaults.

*Why me?*

*What did I do to deserve these horrible things?*

Then, these words came to me while I was on my knees: "I will turn your trauma into your testimony." In that moment, I knew I had a mission. I was ready to receive help. I no longer wanted to die. So, I did the work. I saw many counselors, and my healing happened when I stopped blaming myself and forgiveness became the priority. I took my power back and did not allow my trauma to control me. I lost many people who were close to me. But I will never lose myself again.

# MEET LAKEYDRA HOUSTON

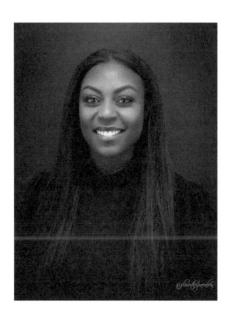

Lakeydra Houston, a US Air Force Veteran and founder of KEY Fit LLC, is deeply committed to enhancing wellness, supporting Veterans, and preventing suicide. Armed with degrees in criminal justice and leadership, she is on a mission to amplify her impact with the added might of a master's in social work, specializing in military and trauma. Certified in ASSIST, victim advocacy, and resiliency training, Lakeydra brings a decade of expertise in addressing domestic violence, sexual assault prevention, and mental health support. Her dedication extends to active community outreach, collaborating with esteemed organizations, such as the Texas Association Against Sexual Assault, American Corporate Partners, Interactive Advocacy, and The Pink Berets, where she serves as the national outreach coordinator.

Lakeydra's personal triumph over adversity drive her mission to connect with youth and the underprivileged, offering education, tools and resources to help empower, prevent and navigate through sexual assault, domestic violence, and other traumatic situations. She has spoken on national platforms, including the Dallas Cowboys Salute to Service, Dateline NBC, the National Crime Victim Law Institute, the Military Influence Conference, and the Army and Air Force Women's Symposium. Lakeydra was recently named as an honoree of the 2024 Presidential Gold Volunteer Service Award.

～

### *Connect with Lakeydra*
**Master Sergeant (Ret.), US Air Force**

*Email: info@keyfitlle.com*
*LinkedIn: Lakeydra Houston*
*Website: www.keyfitlle.com*

～

# Your Turn

What came up for you in this story?

_____
_____
_____
_____
_____
_____
_____
_____
_____
_____
_____
_____
_____
_____
_____
_____
_____
_____
_____
_____
_____
_____
_____
_____
_____

# CHAPTER 17
## CONDUCT UNBECOMING

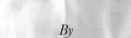

*By*
*Robert "Led" Ledogar*

The call came late in the afternoon on April 20, 2020. My chief, Bryan, sounded pissed. I could hear the verdict in his voice before he even spoke the words. "You were fired." I was speechless. Honestly, as bad as the situation got, I was not expecting that. I actually believed I would survive this ridiculous investigation. I did not want to believe Bryan, but I trusted him like a brother. He quickly forwarded me the email, and there it was in black and white. I, Bobby Ledogar, Supervisory Deputy US Marshal, had been officially fired, removed from the Marshals Service for "conduct unbecoming." In other words, I failed to play along. So, they washed their hands of me. If I'd said nothing about the sexual and physical harassment of Dawn, a gay, female subordinate, if I'd turned a blind eye, I'd still have my job *and* my retirement.

"You've got to fight this, Bobby," Bryan rallied.

*Fight this?!*

A Chief Deputy US Marshal, the designated deciding official, had literally just said, "We don't have the faith or confidence for you to perform at a satisfactory level." If they had only looked at my performance ratings; they would have seen that I consistently performed at an "outstanding" level throughout my career. I had done my job, beyond what was expected. I stood up for the innocent. I confronted the bullies—a handful of federal and local law enforcement officers—and I'd do it again. This was a slap in the face. I wasn't sure I had any more fight left in me. I barely had what it took to break the news to my wife, Roseanne.

After hanging up with Bryan, I shuffled around the house. I lumbered around from room to room—lost, my feet dragging. The words "conduct unbecoming" hanging over my head like a cloud of shame. I had officially been canned from a job that I loved, a job that I was great at and would have given my life for. Instead, I lost all confidence in myself. Had it not been for my good friends believing in me and standing up for me when the chips were down, I don't know what I would have done. To say nothing of my team of lawyers. They all, in their own way, had a hand in keeping me going. I am also thankful for my family and friends. They, too, kept me going. Mostly, I am grateful for Roseanne. She had every right to throw me away, but she never did. She never gave up on me. She believed I did the right thing in protecting Dawn.

The shame and sadness buried me. I was hoping it was all just a bad dream. We were in a worldwide pandemic. The government was shutdown. The Marshals were teleworking, sitting at home, not out on the streets making arrests. I was on leave. I had no cases to work, no court appearances, and no investigations. I had just seventy days to retire, after twenty-five years of service.

I must have read the deciding official's email a hundred times over the next few weeks. That's when I started seeing mistakes. Those small discrepancies were like morsels of hope. I could feel myself getting back into the fight. I became obsessed with finding the holes in the agency's argument, so much so that it put me and Roseanne at odds. We started arguing—a lot! She was over it, ready to close that chapter of our lives. She gave me two weeks to whine and cry about it. I was so depressed. I had no money, no job, no medical insurance. I was applying for work at Home Depot.

*It was rock bottom, and I was angry.*

"Isn't it enough that they stole our peace?!" Roseanne argued. "We can make our money back, but we can never get back our peace."

I was so afraid she was going to leave me because I had failed her. I felt like such a loser. My saving grace was when Roseanne agreed to speak with my lawyers. She was tired of listening to my bitching and bullshit. She needed to hear it from the horse's mouth that we still had a legal leg to stand on. My lawyers laid it all out for her. They answered all of her questions—honestly. Because they still believed I had a case, I began to see a fire rise up in Roseanne. Those who were behind me fanned the flames of her confidence—and mine, too. So many of my colleagues stood in our corner, even after my termination. They knew I did the right thing by standing up for Dawn, trying to protect her from the men in the task force who were harassing her. My good friend and former partner, Craig, combed through every last document and interview from the case, looking for anything that was out of place. Bryan spent hours on the phone with me and Roseanne, talking us off the ledge. Both men were laser focused on keeping us close and safe.

I had good days, and I had bad days. The good days were okay, but the bad days were the worst, ridden with fear, stress, shame, embarrassment, and anxiety. I was always afraid my lead lawyer was going to give up on me. I was waiting for the day he would come to me and say, "We're done. It's over."

When I admitted that to him, he just laughed, and said "Why would you think that?"

You would have to be in my position to understand. When your agency betrays you, it is a lonely place to be—an island. After a while, you start to believe the bad stuff people say about you. It gets under your skin, and it gets harder to see through the lies, especially after the rest of the world goes back to their everyday lives without you. Even those who created the mess had moved on, only they got what I didn't get—closure, an honorable retirement, and pensions.

I was defeated and ashamed—no visible wounds ... only inner demons trying to keep me down. I lost all sense of pride I had in being a Marshal. I no longer felt proud the way my peers feel proud of their service in being a cop, a firefighter or a military serviceman. I lost that feeling, and it sucked. I blame the Marshals for killing that part of me. They knew me. They knew how proud I was to be a part of the agency and how much I loved my job and the men and women I worked with. Roseanne and I welcomed them all into our home. I believed in my work family, but in the end, my leadership did not feel the same way about me. And that sucked more than anything.

A good friend of mine, who also served in the United States Navy and the United States Marshals Service, a true American hero, called me one day not long after I was fired. He got screwed over by the Marshals because he was no tool. His friendship was especially timely; it got me through my own personal dismantling. He told me how he refused to have anything in his home resembling the US Marshals—not one plaque, picture or piece of memorabilia. He said, "I don't even carry my Marshal retirement creds or ID."

When I hung up the phone with him, I sat for a minute or two staring at the wall displaying all my Marshal swag. All the pain, shame and dishonor bubbled up to the surface, threatening to spill over the top. I was angry and upset. After all I had done for the Marshals, nationwide and internationally, they had thrown me away like I was nothing. I stood up and, one by one, I began taking down every plaque, award, photograph, and commendation given to me by the Marshals Service. I shoved all of it into boxes and bags. In doing so, I took my power back. My mother-in-law, Nella, saw what I was doing and went straight to Roseanne. She was concerned by my sudden need to rid myself of these once-important shiny things. Roseanne was unmoved by my behavior and said to her mother, "We are to do nothing."

A few days later, Roseanne came to me and asked, "Are you okay?" She knew who I had spoken with. She knew our history, and she also knew me well enough to know that even if I wasn't okay in that moment, I would be again. The truth is a weight was lifted. It was just stuff taking up space on my walls. It wasn't who or what I am. All that Marshal memorabilia was just bits and pieces of one man's career. That's not what makes a man. What makes a man is what he has on the inside—integrity, strength, determination, courage. Those are things that cannot be boxed up, bagged and/or put away—not even when he's dead. That stuff, nobody can touch.

# MEET ROBERT "BOBBY" LEDOGAR

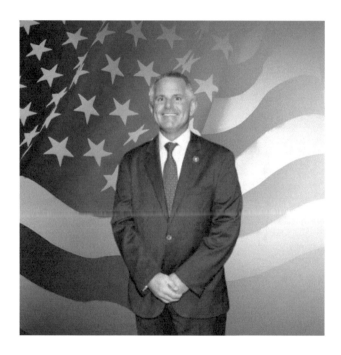

With more than 30 years of military and federal law enforcement experience, Robert "Bobby" Ledogar began his career in the United States Navy as master-at-arms petty officer—military police investigator and instructor. He established himself as a values-based leader, centered on integrity, compassion, community, and respect. As a former Supervisory Deputy US Marshal, reporting to the presidentially appointed US Marshal and Chief Deputy US Marshal, Robert managed missions for the Eastern District of New York, the eighth largest district in the nation. He was directly involved in enforcement, criminal investigations, judiciary and dignitary protection, fugitive apprehension, and prisoner security and handling. He supervised the most diverse unit of men and women and was part of the nation's largest fugitive task force. Robert currently resides in Florida with his wife, Roseanne. He anticipates a 2024 launch of his new book "LED: Being Brooklyn," a detailed account of how he was fired from the US Marshals Service (just 70 days outside of his retirement) for honoring his professional oath and strong Brooklyn upbringing.

～

### Connect with Bobby
**US Navy, US Marshals Service & Veteran Affairs Healthcare (Ret.)**

*Email: rled26@aol.com*
*LinkedIn: Robert Ledoger*
*Website: www.LEDBeingBrooklyn.com*

～

# Your Turn

What came up for you in this story?

_____
_____
_____
_____
_____
_____
_____
_____
_____
_____
_____
_____
_____
_____
_____
_____
_____
_____
_____
_____
_____
_____
_____

# CHAPTER 18
# ADDICTION: THE ANTITHETICAL GIFT

By
*Mike Peyton*

Wearing the proverbial "scarlet letter," despite never having been convicted of a crime and having a spotless record my entire life, had a profound impact on me. How can people automatically presume an individual is guilty of a crime without evidence, examination of witnesses, and diligently, if not objectively utilizing their discernment on both sides of the narrative? I realize this isn't the optimal mindset or the best series of questions to ask. It wasn't until I completely surrendered to my Maker that my mental and spiritual apertures truly opened. Amidst the trials, I am thriving "because greater is He that is in me than he that is in the world." *

While sitting idly in my jail cell, I asked myself a couple of

---

\* 1 John 4:4 New King James Version

critical questions: *Why is this happening to me, and what mistakes did **I** make along the way that cultivated my current predicament?* These two questions opened Pandora's box for self-enlightenment and the dawn of another transformational phase in my life.

A twenty-year career in the SEAL Teams allowed me to see and experience various regions of the world, from war-torn and uncertain to first-world societies outside of the United States. Furthermore, the Teams trained and equipped me to operate in less-than-ideal circumstances, where the odds could shift at the drop of a hat. The Teams have a brilliant way of preparing operators to protect western constructs, and I am forever grateful to have served with some of the most heroic and patriotic individuals this country has to offer.

Toward the end of my career, I went through a contentious divorce—a battle the Teams did not prepare me for. In the process, I filed for bankruptcy, foreclosed on my house, agreed to a lop-sided custody arrangement, and picked up the bottle after five years of abstinence: terrible choice! I wrestled with alcohol my entire teen and adult life. It was the mistress that kept plunging and securing its hooks in me, despite my attempts of eradication. With certainty, I can say that at least 95 percent of my personal and professional quandaries correlate back to this persistent and invasive tyrant. A couple more years with this chaotic impostor at the helm brought me to a life-altering decision point—either go to rehab and evict this monster or lose the remainder of my accumulated scraps and die. In my despair, I petitioned the Lord in conviction that if He delivered me from this wicked oppressor, I would earnestly work for Him. Three days later, I was detoxing at the Naval Hospital in San Diego. Without question, this was a providential act with my brother advocating the entire way and moving mountains to make it happen.

Upon completion of rehab, I was adamant about helping

other operators wrestling with this problem. After retiring from the Navy, I founded a nonprofit organization focused on addiction recovery. The mission was faith-oriented with a holistic approach to combat this Goliath. The foundation's modalities encompassed healing of the entire person (body, mind, and spirit). Programs are tailored to individual needs. The foundation's board, partners, and service providers were building the plane as it was flying, which was an amazing feat.

One fundamental tenet in most recovery programs is to not make any major life-altering decisions within the first year of sobriety. I carried the burden of four—two of my own volition. Because I was still active duty and in a recovery program, the Navy cut orders back to Virginia, where I spent majority of my career, right up to the remainder of it. In hindsight, this was a good call because I was familiar with the area, had a support network of friends and family, and it allowed me a twilight tour prior to retiring. Four months into this transition and still thinking with a drunk brain, I ended a long-distance relationship with an amazing human being of a woman and immediately jumped headfirst into a new romantic relationship.

My childhood trauma and the fear of being alone massively outweighed all of the blatant warning signs my new partner revealed about herself. It appeared I had attracted yet another woman within the "Cluster B" category of personality disorders. I reasoned and justified to myself that it would be different this time because I have the resources to help her (and me), whereas I didn't in my prior relationships with this particular type of personality. I just knew that we would get to the root as to why we were consistently having up to ten-plus hours of nonsensical, circular arguments and sleepless nights—her hair-trigger reactions, the gaslighting and "splitting," our traumas, my addiction and avoidant attachment style, and her extreme fear of abandonment.

*As a couple, we were a fool's errand, indeed.*

Two and a half years of this toxic relationship was plenty, and it was time to end it—permanently. I had "ended" it multiple times before, but this time the suicide threats and the stalking wouldn't persuade me to come back. I had recently obtained custody of my son, and I could not bring him into an unstable environment like that; enough was enough. Being diagnosed with cancer didn't hold a candle to the terror this relationship caused me.

I had just graduated from Harvard's flagship Executive Education Program—Professional Leadership Development, was recovering from cancer surgery, and was fully determined to take the foundation to the next level—or two. Ten days later, the first criminal charge of malicious wounding came for me.

The frigid holding cell smelled like urine. Clearly, it had made a permanent home in the pores of the aging reinforced concrete. At a snail-like pace, the minutes turned into hours, and I began to question whether or not this was going to be a "process and release" for me. I looked around at the others who were gracing their presence in this dystopic nightmare. Never having experienced this before, I imagined they were the typical crew of misfits: three street hooligans, a couple of drunks, and a shirtless three-hundred pound man laying belly-up on the floor, biting his hand until he drew blood and occasionally wiping his feces on the wall.

*At last!*

The corrections officer summoned me to appear in front of the magistrate. My hands and feet were shackled for escort. With indifference, the magistrate explained that she could not release me due to the egregious nature of the charge and that I must stay in jail to await a bond hearing. The truths that surfaced from Stanford's Prison experiment began to surface during the in-take process. I was guilty in their eyes, despite not actually being convicted of a crime. Mugshot, fingerprints, DNA swab, and the cavity/strip search is standard (and necessary) protocol to reside in this house of horror. After this subhuman experience, and unbeknownst to me, I was marching towards a pod that held the hardened inmates. These inmates were either charged and/or convicted of serious crimes and most of them had a fathom-long criminal record.

I was as green as they came in this system. One of the only prison movies I ever watched was Shawshank Redemption. I wrote a paper in college on recidivism and drug crimes. This was the extent of my criminal justice knowledge. With God's grace, I retained an impeccable defense attorney and a week later had my first bond hearing.

Standing shackled in front of the judge with my brother and sister in the courtroom pews, my attorney and the prosecutor went at it for a good ten minutes. The judge listened intently to both arguments, then she set the bond for $5,000 with no stipulations. Immediately, the prosecutor objected and appealed the decision. As charges kept trickling in, I ended up having four more bond hearings because the prosecution continued to appeal the various judge's approved decisions. After the fifth, there were no more appeals, and I finished my jail stent after thirty-one days. Despite living in perdition, God used me as a beacon of light with Bible studies for those who wanted to participate, including prayer groups. My "cellie" gave his life to Christ.

*Glory to God!*

Through these trials by fire and blessed with a four-year sober mind, I have retained many invaluable lessons and will share four that have continual resonance: Firstly, there are two personifications an individual can choose to emulate, either the Machiavellian archetype filled with hate, discontent, malice, and vengeance or the Christ-like archetype, encompassing virtue, forgiveness, love, and humility. Secondly, never quit, despite the opposition. Remember, it's okay to take a pause in order to recalibrate, refocus, and realign. But don't quit doing the right thing, regardless of temporal circumstances, like a tarnished reputation or getting stripped of material goods. Persevere to the end because this is part of the self-actualization, refinement, and purification process, which is significantly more valuable. Thirdly, do not make any major life-altering decisions within the first year of sobriety. Trust me on this one. And lastly, don't make decisions with a fear-driven mindset. This is a set-up for failure at all levels and in every capacity. Instead, counter this determined intruder with knowledge, understanding, and faith.

# MEET MICHAEL PEYTON

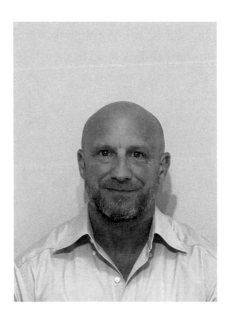

Born a Wyoming native and raised in Tucson Arizona's Sonoran Desert, Michael Peyton enlisted in the United States Navy with the high achievement of becoming a Navy SEAL. After 21 years of service that included four deployments to Afghanistan and two to Iraq, he retired with a strong willingness to share his acumen and aptitude with those who would like to further develop and refine their own purpose.

Even in childhood, Mike understood the SEAL Teams were purposeful in recruiting exclusively from a circle of men who had the fortitude and will to fulfill the physical and mental demand, which is why he fought so valiantly to cope with and overcome adversity throughout his life, including a battle with cancer. Mike's newfound passion is to mentor and lead both individuals and teams triumphantly through life's minefield, exploring both positive and negative paradigms and always doing so through an empathetic lens.

∽

### Connect with Mike
*Navy SEAL (Ret.), Empath, Aspiring Author*

*Email: michaelpeyton239@gmail.com*

∽

# Your Turn

What came up for you in this story?

_____
_____
_____
_____
_____
_____
_____
_____
_____
_____
_____
_____
_____
_____
_____
_____
_____
_____
_____
_____
_____
_____
_____
_____
_____
_____
_____
_____

# CHAPTER 19
# A ROOKIE COP'S LONGEST RIDE

—⌣∞⌣—

*By*

*Richard T. Oakley*

My story began six months out of the academy as a twenty-four-year-old rookie, a patrolman in New Brunswick, New Jersey. It's a story that haunted me throughout my thirty-year law enforcement career. The trauma I endured changed the way that I looked at things, people, and life.

June 14, 1968 started off as a typical workday. I reported to headquarters at 0530. Upon reporting to briefing, we were informed of the events from the previous shift and handed our assignments. I was assigned to patrol—Southside sector. During my tour, I responded to several calls for service—typical stuff. I recall the day being uneventful. After my tour ended, I left headquarters and drove to my apartment. When I got home, I removed my duty belt and uniform shirt. Still in my work trousers, I remembered forgetting to pick something up from the store, so I got into my 1965 Ford Mustang and headed out. I noticed three caucasian males standing in my complex. I knew these individuals had criminal records from previous encounters. I decided to make contact to determine why they were in this area. I pulled up to where they were standing and questioned them; at which point, two of the males pulled pistols on me, forcing me into the back seat of my own vehicle. One of the males took the driver's seat. One sat in the passenger seat, holding a weapon on me. The third guy got in the back seat with me. My heart was pounding. I felt lightheaded. My palms were sweating. I knew this was my end.

As we drove away, the driver turned on the radio to the local news. That's when I heard these men were wanted for armed robbery. They robbed a Florsheim shoe store at gunpoint and fled to my neighborhood. As soon as they heard the news account, they all looked to see my reaction. That's when the threats began. One of the men said, "You should have minded your own business."

I remained silent. I didn't want to anger them. The driver stopped to pick up a black female named Jeanie. She was the girlfriend of one of the men. I noticed we were headed toward Trenton, up Route 22 East, and then toward New York City. When we left New Jersey, I heard one of them say, "We're going for broke." They had violated the Lindberg Law, the act making kidnapping a federal offense, allowing federal investigators the authority to pursue kidnappers across state jurisdictions. The men spoke often of killing me and dumping me along the road.

I thought about my two young sons. What would happen to them? Would they be alright? How would my mom, younger brother, and sister take it? I could feel the rapid pulse throbbing in my neck. My breathing was labored. I had no hope of getting out alive. I was asked if I had a family. I was asked their names. I told the men that I was married with two young sons. One of the men said he would go after my family if I ratted on them.

We arrived in New York City at the intersection of 72nd Street and West End Avenue. The three men and the young woman exited my car and got lost in the crowded street. I sat frozen in my vehicle for a long time, wondering why they decided to let me go. When I returned to New Brunswick, I went to my sergeant's home to inform him what had happened. My sergeant asked me if I was armed.

"Yes," I replied.

That response haunted me for a long time because I wasn't armed, but I knew that department regulations required officers to carry their gun and badge off duty. I was afraid of what would happen to me if I'd told the truth. This was my dream job. I had only been on six months. My sergeant contacted the chief, the deputy chief, and the New York City Police Department. We were told to go to the NYPD's 20th precinct, the area where I was dropped off. So, I drove back to New York City that evening with my sergeant, chief of detectives, and a lieutenant from the Middlesex County Prosecutor's Office. We met with three detectives who questioned me about the kidnapping. The NYPD put out a Be on the Lookout (BOLO) for the three men. I knew it was going to be a long night. I provided descriptions of the four suspects. My adrenaline was working overtime. After questioning, I was shown a cot for the night. I futilely tried sleeping with the events of the day fluttering through my mind and the noise of a very active precinct.

Several days later, two of the three men were located and arrested in a flop house in Manhattan. They were taken to a court in New York to be prosecuted and prepared for extradition and transport to a municipal court in New Jersey for arraignment and bail hearing. Bail was set for $25,000 each. The other two suspects and the girlfriend remained at large until July 27, 1968, when they were all apprehended.

On February 4, 1969, the jury selection process began. Finding an impartial jury was not an easy task because of the lack of popularity for the police at the time. The next day, the jurors were given instructions by the presiding judge, explaining their role and what evidence would be considered. After the jurors were presented with opening statements, I was called to the witness stand and administered the oath. That oath stayed with me forever.

I was asked to recount the kidnapping through a series of questions by the prosecutor. The defense team took notes and the three men who held me at gunpoint and drove me across state lines watched on. I was on the witness stand for several hours. It was not easy to maintain my composure.

After lunch, the cross-examination began, an attempt to conjure reasonable doubt. I was shaking. My chest heaved. My hands were sweaty, and I felt like someone had kicked me in the gut. Each of the three defense attorneys cross-examined me, attempting to get me to admit that I wasn't kidnapped but rather went along for a ride because I was interested in the black female, Jeanie. He hammered away at that story. I lost it a few times because I knew better. The cross-examination was grueling and intense. I was emotionally drained. One of the defense attorneys got me to confess that I was *not* armed, even though I testified during direct examination that I had my duty weapon on me. I was still a probationary officer. I was afraid of losing my job because of the department rule requiring off-duty officers to carry, so I initially lied to my sergeant and to the court.

Once my cross-examination was complete, one of the men was called to the witness stand. His attorney asked him what happened on June 14, 1968. He replied, "We did not kidnap Mr. Oakley. He came with us willingly because he liked Jeanie." He also said that they knew I was a cop and that I didn't have a gun. "We would never kidnap a cop," he said.

By the time closing arguments took place, I had lost hope in the case.

On February 8, 1969, the judge gave the jury deliberation instructions. He informed them that the decision had to be unanimous. The jury was then returned to the room to begin deliberations. At 5:00 p.m., the jury was allowed to go home for the evening. The next day, the jury returned and continued their deliberations. After three hours, the jurors had reached a verdict. My adrenaline kicked in. I nervously watched the jurors enter the courtroom and take their seats in the jury box. The judge asked if they had reached a verdict.

"Yes, your Honor."

The verdict came back—not guilty.

This was the second worst day of my life. I was disappointed and drained. I left the courtroom, got into my car, and cried. I went straight to the local bar and drank for several hours. My friends tried consoling me. When I got home, I didn't want to talk to anyone. That day, I began my descent into heavy drinking. I was a functioning alcoholic. There was no counseling or resources available to deal with such trauma. We were expected to suck it up and move on. So, I lived with the trauma from the kidnapping and the "not-guilty" verdict for years. However, I did not allow it to defeat me. I tell people facing similar trauma to tell the truth, no matter the consequences. I tell them to share their story in a safe space and often. That is the way to healing, and I am here to tell you, "Believe in yourself. Focus on your mental and physical health. Tune out the noise, and don't be distracted by your critic. Remember, you are important." I wish I'd had someone to give me, the twenty-four-year-old rookie police officer in 1968, that same advice.

# MEET RICH OAKLEY

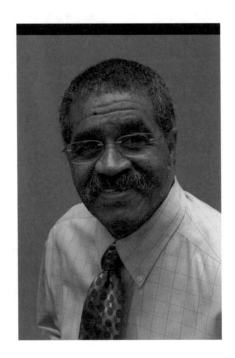

Before joining the DEA in 1974, Richard T. Oakley was a police officer in New Brunswick, New Jersey. He joined the department on September 10, 1967. After graduating from the New Jersey State Police Academy, Rich was assigned to the patrol division and was later promoted to the rank of detective, assigned to the Narcotics Bureau. Rich has 30 years of law enforcement experience, 23 of which were spent with the Drug Enforcement Administration (DEA) in positions that included: special agent in the New York Field Division, special agent in the Newark Field Division, division training coordinator (Newark, New Jersey), and supervisory special agent in the San Francisco Field Division. He also served at the DEA Headquarters in Arlington, Virginia as staff coordinator for the Policy and Procedures Unit, special assistant to the deputy administrator for Operations, special assistant to the DEA administrator, executive secretary of the DEA Career Board, and finally retiring as assistant special agent in charge. Rich's career culminated in several significant drug operations, which led to many awards, commendations, and proclamations for his service.

∾

### Connect with Rich
**DEA Senior Special Agent (Ret.)**

*Email: jurassicnarc@gmail.com*

∾

# Your Turn

What came up for you in this story?

_____
_____
_____
_____
_____
_____
_____
_____
_____
_____
_____
_____
_____
_____
_____
_____
_____
_____
_____
_____
_____
_____
_____
_____
_____

# CHAPTER 20
# THE WISDOM OF FORGIVENESS

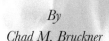

*By*
*Chad M. Bruckner*

I n February 2008, thirty months after serving in Iraq, I was
hired as a police officer. I remember standing in my suit, my
new bride next to me. Kristen and I were married just five
months earlier. She held the Bible in her hand, while I listened
intently to the mayor read the creed in a public session. Council
members sat behind me. The chief of police stood inches away.
How could I have known then that the creed I swore an oath to
would betray me?

It was a happy night—glorious. My parents, in-laws, siblings,
and grandparents were in attendance. I breezed right through
field training. My FTO remarked that no one had gone through
the program with such ease. I was twenty-seven years old, and I
had combat experience. I served eight years in the US Army as
an infantry leader. I was nearly killed in Iraq while leading

combat missions. However, I didn't recognize my own self-confidence in those early days as an officer.

In my thirteen-year career, I was a great police officer. After much reflection, I can say that with peace and confidence. I have a huge heart. I cared a great deal, and I was exceptional in my role. I developed high-value relationships, not only with members of my agency but surrounding agencies as well. I became a resource for other cops. I'm the guy who would give my last few dollars to a stranger in need over my own kids because my children know we'll be okay in the end. Helping brings me a sense of purpose. I love people and enjoy meeting them where they are in life, and that is not always easy. I have held the dead and injured in my arms, including children. I would do every bit of it again, even the bad stuff because it is all a part of the package of human service. But it comes at a cost.

My third year on, there was an opening for detective. I was ready. I had proven myself to be a top performer on the street. However, I was passed over for a female officer who did not work nearly as hard. The chief disclosed to me that I was the more qualified candidate, but he was going to promote the other officer. He assured me my time would come. I had a front row seat to politics over people. I was confused about this promotion "process." Plus, watching the newly promoted detective underperform in her daily duties only lowered my self-esteem.

*Was merit not the standard?*

Nevertheless, I pressed on, committing myself to service. One year later, I was chomping at the bit for more opportunities to serve. But there were no more detective openings. So, I did what any determined young cop who cares about his community would do. I created my own detective division and pitched it to the chief. I called it the Street Crimes Unit (SCU). It was my take on fixing our community's open-air drug market. The chief embraced it. I worked this unit for one month alone without any supervision, then my partner, Nick, joined me from patrol. Together, the two of us spent a lot of time cleaning up the streets. An ambitious patrol sergeant took notice and began his climb to become our supervisor.

Over time, we had a lot of success, arresting more than 250 felony drug dealers, violent offenders, and people negatively affecting the quality of life in town. The Street Crimes Unit reduced crime by 40 percent. It was incredible! While in the military, I had been a part of some successful operations but nothing like this. I literally smiled as I fell asleep because of the positive impact we were having. If only I could have bottled up that feeling and saved it for later.

Here's the thing about success. It can create monsters. The ambitious patrol sergeant schemed and found a way to remove the existing detective sergeant from his position, so he could take over. He became my first line supervisor, and he would use this position for personal gain. With every arrest we made, the ambitious sergeant, once sitting on the periphery, was now getting accolades for the work my partner and I were doing. His sphere of influence grew, and I was perfectly fine with that. After all, we were a team. We were supposed to work together and rise together.

After working with this sergeant every day for seven years, having been exposed to his secrets and soul, I saw a broken man. He was no team player and seemed to enjoy hurting others to make himself feel better. For example, he once denied my request for a bereavement day when my wife, Kristen, suffered an ectopic miscarriage. He suggested I use a vacation day instead. I was confused, so I went over his head to the chief. I filed a complaint. This was a difficult time for me and Kristen, and I couldn't process my first line supervisor working against me. The chief admonished him, and the sergeant offered an apology. It was another lesson in dealing with broken men within a broken system. Truth: I was broken, too. But I would have happily used a vacation day so that I could be present with me wife. My issue was that this ambitious sergeant created an unfair system; the rules were different depending on who was playing.

In 2019, eleven years into my policing career, I got so low I began having suicidal ideations. I contemplated ending my life ... ending my pain. I couldn't see a path forward, and the hopelessness led to great despair. I told my wife I thought about driving my car off an overpass. I was scared and emotional. Being betrayed by my own organization was brutal. I gave so much of myself to that agency. I forged meaningful relationships. I matured and grew on a personal level because of it. It was literally my second home. Betrayal that comes from within one's own police department is a hurt that cannot be put into words. It's been several years since my incident, and I'm still working through it.

You see, that ambitious sergeant later became my chief, and within eighteen months, I was back on patrol. I did not request this assignment. That decision was made on the heels of a complaint made against him for the way in which he administered the promotional process. The whole department signed the memo, and me and my partner, being the most outspoken, paid the price for it. In all my years in public service —military and law enforcement—I never had disciplinary issues. Sure, I made mistakes, but I was always professional. This move was personal, and everyone knew it.

The anger I felt was unbearable. I couldn't sleep. I wanted vengeance. I felt I had little control over my life. The besiege of negativity was too much. Anger and insecurity took over during the day. Anxiety and fear ruled the night. I began drinking to mask the pain and shame. I developed such a hatred and resentment for public service, I began to see everyone as a fake and phony. It wasn't fair to label everyone that way, but I had had enough.

After thirteen years, I submitted my notice to retire and was gone three weeks later. It was a painful exit—no exit interview, no one from the municipality asked questions. I had given so much to my community. I paid an emotional and mental price to keep them safe. I missed family events. It's what service required, and I was left feeling like a giant fool. So, I did what fools do—tuck tail and run. I was hurting, nearing burnout. I was a ticking time bomb. At home, I would excuse myself to the basement to sit in solitude with a four-pack to self-medicate my sorrows. I would wake the next morning with a masked smile. It hid my true feelings. The shame was real, like nothing I'd ever felt before. I was not equipped to properly identify the shame; and that was dangerous. Someone told me, "Don't let them know they won. Keep it inside."

*That was the worst advice!*

I was struggling to pick up the pieces. I was no longer a cop. I would have to find new ways to serve. It was a challenge. My wife, Kristen, reminded me of the important mission ahead. "You have a beautiful family who loves you and looks to you for leadership," she said. "Our kids think the world of you. Isn't that enough?"

Asking for help was the greatest gift I gave myself. I had so much to lose and so many loving relationships. I can't believe I ever thought of ending my life. I still have so much to contribute, and yet my light was almost extinguished. That won't happen again.

My second greatest gift was to forgive, learning to move on and grow from the pain. Forgiveness requires a lot of work, time, and emotion. But I remain committed to forgiving my former chief. Forgiveness, ultimately, serves the soul, setting an example for others in a broken world.

# MEET CHAD BRUCKNER

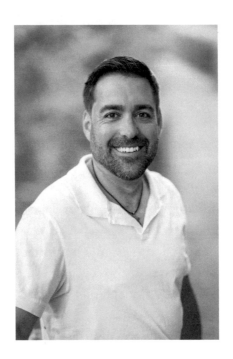

Chad Bruckner, retired Pennsylvania police detective and combat Veteran, served 13 years in law enforcement and eight years in the United States Army. Today, he is a small business owner, professional speaker, coach, and humanitarian. Chad holds a master's degree in digital forensics and is a certified recovery specialist. As a coach, his aim is to help individuals and organizations reach their full potential in performance and morale, beginning with a balanced, holistic, and healthy lifestyle.

## *Connect with Chad*

*Performance Coach, Speaker, Police Officer & Army Veteran*

*Author of The Holy Trinity of Successful and Healthy Police Organizations: Improving*

*Leadership, Culture and Wellness*

*Email: chadmotivates@gmail.com*

*Website: https://motivate-change.com/*

# Your Turn

What came up for you in this story?

_____
_____
_____
_____
_____
_____
_____
_____
_____
_____
_____
_____
_____
_____
_____
_____
_____
_____
_____
_____
_____
_____
_____
_____
_____
_____
_____
_____

# CHAPTER 21
# UNPACKING MY EMOTIONAL RUCKSACK

*By*
*Daniel Torrez*

## BEFORE THE BADGE

At an early age, I wanted to become a police officer or a firefighter. This was a result of regularly watching 1970's cop shows and the television series Emergency! Despite growing up in a middle-class, Roman Catholic family, I felt my dream slipping away due to my affinity for finding trouble as a teenager. On track to becoming a fifth-year senior, it took me five years plus summer school to graduate.

Ultimately, a positive police encounter during a "beer run" solidified my goal of becoming a police officer. I enlisted in the Army at the age of seventeen to serve my country and gain law enforcement experience. I was proud to follow in the footsteps of my dad and brother by serving in the military.

On July 12, 1985, I was at home with my mom, dad, and younger sister. While in the shower, I heard my mom yelling and knocking on the door. My gut told me that something had happened to my dad. He had recently decided to leave the hospital to be with his family, despite his cancer prognosis. Hurriedly, I dried off, put on some clothes, and went to my parents' bedroom where I found my dad unresponsive; he had quietly passed away. I had to be there for my mom and younger sister while notifying my brothers that our dad was gone.

I could have canceled my enlistment because of my dad's cancer. I chose not to, based on a conversation I had with him two weeks before he passed. He told me he believed in me and that he was proud of me. He also said, "A Torrez never quits." After the ambulance took my dad away, I went to my parents' bedroom and felt engulfed in the stench of death. It's a very distinct smell when cancer has eaten away at the body. I would experience this stench a few more times in the Army.

I didn't cry when my dad passed away or at his funeral four days later. I was too angry. I was ready to "Be All You Can Be." I left home three weeks later for Fort McClellan, Alabama. Advanced training taught me what it took to be a great MP— don't let things get to you and show no emotion. I could never have imagined what an expert I would become at stuffing my emotions into my rucksack.

## BEHIND THE BADGE

My first duty station was Fort Hood, Texas. I immersed myself in becoming *the* best MP I could be. I volunteered for training, learning from both great and bad leaders. The old timers made it seem "normal" to hit the bars after duty and stay out all night, regardless of when they had to report for duty. I was reacting negatively and not responding appropriately to the trauma I experienced. Alcohol became my crutch, along with high-risk behaviors, fighting, and off-duty conduct that pushed the limit.

It was the stench of death from my first medical emergency call that took me back to my parents' bedroom. I arrived before the paramedics to find a young mother screaming, "Save my baby!" The woman's fourteen-year-old daughter was on the couch, surrounded by the stench of death. I knew in my heart she had passed. She was pale and cold to the touch. Leukemia took her. To put the mother at ease, I moved the girl onto the carpet and began CPR. Relieved, she said, "Thank you for saving my baby!"

The paramedics arrived and looked at me, as if to say, *What are you doing? She's gone?* As I glanced toward the mother, they understood and took over CPR. I turned in my report and got a "Good job!" from the desk sergeant.

In 1986, there were no debriefs or "How are you doing?" So, the trauma from that incident, the death of a fellow MP, and other critical incidents were stuffed into my rucksack with my emotions. The anger, drinking, fighting, and high-risk behaviors were steadily mounting. I asked my leadership for help but received little. Many of my senior leaders had served in Vietnam. They followed the SUDO concept: Suck it up and drive on!

Still trying to grieve, I asked the one person I knew who could help me, a Catholic chaplain. I poured my heart out with anticipation of some priestly guidance. Instead, he handed me a pamphlet and told me to read it.

*Strike one!*

I threw the pamphlet away, and it was business as usual. A few months later, I sought help again. This time, he handed me a book on how to grieve the loss of a loved one.

*Strike two!*

No need to ask for help a third time. My trajectory was set, I would suppress my emotions and "Be All I Could Be!" I followed this trajectory throughout my twenty-one year Army career that involved many more critical incidents, including traffic fatalities, drownings, dismembered bodies, humanitarian/disaster relief, United Nations Peacekeeping, and combat operations.

~

## AFTER THE BADGE

After retiring from the Army, I returned home to Phoenix and began working with the Arizona Department of Corrections. My grant-funded position was to help develop a restorative justice program. The Victim Offender Dialogue (VOD) program brought victims of violent crime face-to-face with their offender. I conducted several successful dialogues, primarily with homicide and sex offense victims.

As the new grant cycle approached, I was eager to help give victims a voice they had not had before, as they navigated their journey toward healing. Regrettably, someone in my agency did not seek renewal of my position. This decision was made in April of 2020, but I did not find out until late July. It was a huge gut punch that completely took my breath away. I was in a state of controlled aggression. Could I stuff these feelings in my rucksack on top of all the trauma from the previous thirty-five years?

I told my lovely wife I would be unemployed as of October 1st. I think she was even more outraged than me. I didn't feel I was mentally ready to stay with the agency, so I began looking for a new job. I felt shame and disappointment as I was not going to be able to provide for my family. I was in a dark place and in a downward spiral. Alcohol became my crutch again, and I thought to myself, *This could all end if ...*

I never did complete that thought, and it never entered my mind again, thanks to my lovely wife for having my back and reassuring me that we would be okay. Revitalized with the intestinal fortitude to move forward, I realized I had been in much worse situations. I took another role in a different department and am grateful for the few executive leaders who offered support throughout my transition.

The situation had such a profound effect on me, I decided to seek additional support. In October 2021, I found The Power of Our Story, a platform whose mainstay is connection and non-judgmental support. In sharing my story, I allowed myself to be vulnerable. I felt my emotional rucksack emptying, as I began my journey of self-discovery. Being a part of this tribe helped me seek mental health support. I began therapy in June 2022 and was diagnosed with PTSD. My vulnerability became my strength; it feeds my resilience. I reclaimed my identity and lost the persona I was clinging to since graduating from Ranger School. I realized it was okay to be Daniel vs. "Ranger Torrez." Ranger Torrez is a part of me, but it's not who I am. I am a husband, father, servant leader, Combat Veteran, and advocate.

After presenting my story at a 1st responder conference, a young firefighter asked what would have helped change my trajectory as a young MP. Life may have been different had the chaplain listened without judgment and offered support. It has been a long road to self-discovery and accepting my PTSD diagnosis. I decided to "disable the label" and continue to be vulnerable. I developed my own way of continuing to prevail. I call it the **AAR/R** method: *Accept, Acknowledge, Respond Appropriately*, and **Reach Out** *when needed*. I applied it as I emerged from the darkness and downward spiral. I had to *AAR/R* my dad's death. I accepted it, acknowledging the impact he had on my life and responding appropriately by sharing both his story and mine. It took reaching out to The Power of Our Story and seeking mental health support.

The ability to seek support is possible at any stage of one's career. My trajectory may have changed if the young MP in me would have sought support, even after the chaplain failed. If you are experiencing job-related trauma, it is never too early or too late to seek support. This is especially true when you are living out your childhood dream, like I was.

# MEET DANIEL TORREZ

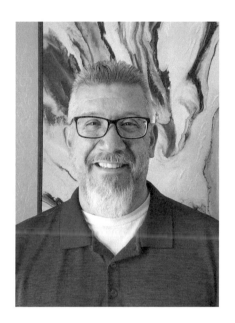

Daniel Torrez, Deputy Director with the National Center for Victims of Crime, helped establish the first Victim Offender Dialogue (VOD) program in Arizona, conducting several dialogues and experiencing firsthand the restorative justice and healing effect on all participants. Daniel served 21 years as a military police officer in the US Army and participated in humanitarian/disaster relief efforts, United Nations Peacekeeping and combat operations. He served as a patrol supervisor, victims advocate, SRT (SWAT) member, non-lethal weapons instructor, master trainer, and was a member of the 3rd US Infantry, The Old Guard. Daniel has also served as a federal law enforcement officer and university director of public safety. He holds a master's degree from Webster University, a bachelor's degree, and certified public manager designation from Arizona State University. He currently lives in Phoenix, Arizona with his lovely wife, Melissa, their cat Sadie, and their dog Ares (the Dog of War).

∿

### Connect with Daniel
*Husband, Father, Servant Leader, Combat Veteran, Advocate*

*LinkedIn: Daniel Torrez, MA, CPM*

∿

# Your Turn

What came up for you in this story?

_____
_____
_____
_____
_____
_____
_____
_____
_____
_____
_____
_____
_____
_____
_____
_____
_____
_____
_____
_____
_____
_____
_____
_____
_____

# CHAPTER 22
# THE LAST TO ABANDON

*By*

*Christopher Hoyer*

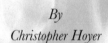

Abandonment can do some serious damage to the human spirit. How do I know? I was born in Portsmouth, New Hampshire in 1969 to a single, black mother. I am told my biological father is white, a United States Marine who was shipped out to the Vietnam War before I made my entrance into the world. He may or may not know that I exist. I sometimes think about what it would be like to meet him, to see if I inherited his ears, his height, and his yearning to serve. I may never know.

Before I could walk, my mom married another man. He took me in as his own. Two years later, he bailed. My mom and I were on our own again. I guess things got too hard for her because she kicked me out of the house when I was fourteen years old. She sent me to live with my stepfather. At eighteen, just as I was gaining some stability, he booted me out of the house over breakfast. He asked, "Do you have your rent money?"

The answer was no, and I became a homeless, high school dropout with nowhere to go. It was snowing outside. I lived in my beat-up car for a while. I got a job, saved up some money, and was finally able to get my own apartment, which my mom moved into for a while. I was in a new town, spending time with the girl I thought I would marry. Things were looking up. I followed the girl across country to Arizona. Six weeks later, she bailed. I was heartbroken—crushed, crying, and discarded once again.

In time, I recovered. I was back on my feet, dating a single mom with a one-year-old daughter. I fell in love with the little girl and married her mother—probably not the best reason for getting married. I just wanted to be a responsible family man, something I didn't see a whole lot of growing up. I wanted to be there for that little girl.

I found my purpose as a street cop. For twenty years, it was my dream job until it wasn't. There was a gunfight, an ambush that cost the life of a fellow officer and forced me to take a life—my fourth as things went. At that point, I had been on the job for eighteen years, having experienced multiple critical incidents, including three officer-involved shootings. I buried sixteen of my brothers, all of whom were killed in the line of duty over the course of my career. By this point, I had two grown children and a wife who was living in my house but wanted nothing to do with me. I was living alone, separated, and on my way to divorce—nearing a meltdown.

One year following the gunfight, after months of counseling and therapy, my department abandoned me. When I dedicated my life to my profession, I really didn't know what I was in for. That never mattered to me because I loved it! I loved it so much that I gave more than 100-percent of myself to the cause. After my buddy was murdered in front of me, I was struggling with the idea of going back to the street. I went to the executive chief officer and said, "Sir, in nineteen years, I have never asked for help. I am asking now, and you are turning your back on me."

The X-O knew it was true, and at my request, he did not insult me with a piss-poor excuse. I was faced with returning to the street, knowing full well I was no longer capable. I was given the option to sign paperwork that would list me as mentally unfit for duty—professional suicide. I did *not* sign on *that* dotted line —no way!

Instead, I took my chances with the criminal element on the street. It didn't go well. My first year was a blur. There were lots of triggers—some good, some bad. If that weren't bad enough, there was the initial investigation of the gunfight and then, of course, attending Police Week in 2017 in honor of the fallen officer from a scene that I had been sent to scout out.

*It was a nightmare!*

I was living alone, no family around for support. Another law enforcement buddy of mine was killed in a major critical incident. My best friend lost his dog in a deployment on my 20th anniversary. My squad mates and my leadership had lost trust in my ability. I had plenty doubts of my own. At one point, I was literally tasked with scraping the barbeque grill at the station because I couldn't be trusted with anything else. Life could not have gotten worse. So, how on Earth was I able to pull out of that tailspin with such a positive outlook on life? How did I survive a life fraught with abandonment issues? It's simple really.

*I CHOOSE to be okay.*

I understand now that my circumstances are not always in my control. Equally as important …not my fault. I learned that as a homeless kid and a storied street cop. So, I let the ownership remain with those whose life decisions impacted me negatively— my biological father, my mother, the girl I traveled across the country with, the woman I married, my department, the twenty-year-old kid who killed an officer and forced my hand, and you get the idea. If they come to me with guilt or shame, I forgive them. If they do not, I simply remember happier times, and I let them go—forgiven.

Today, my life is epic! I went to great lengths to survive my law enforcement career, my marriage, my childhood. I purposefully sought help. I followed through with it, and now I see the beauty life has to offer. I take time to appreciate it whenever I can. When I deliberately chose this path forward, life (in all its fullness) began to unfold before me. Looking back, it occurs to me that as a child, I had little to no say about where I lived, who was in my life, and who cared for me. As a subordinate to my employer, I had little to no say about my career path following one of the worst days of my life. As a father, whose own daughter has stopped talking to me since the divorce, I have zero say about my involvement in her life and the life of my granddaughter.

*I cannot make people love me.*

I could spend a lifetime trying, but I would simply rather speak my peace and keep moving forward with purpose and forgiveness in my heart. The only thing worse than being abandoned, is begging someone to stay. For what it's worth and for whatever reason people in my life leave me, I forgive them. Again, I know it was not my fault. I refuse to sulk and chase after people who, as much as they matter to me, do not have enough love and respect for me to give me a chance to love them the way I know I can and want to. I like to believe I earned it. I am not perfect, but I do my best every day to be a good man. That is to say, I can sleep at night, and I can still look myself in the mirror. I have enough respect for myself to move away from where I am not wanted.

In doing so, I met and fell head over heels for a woman who loves me unconditionally and who, I know in my heart, will never abandon me. She is my best friend! Just the other day, I knelt down on one knee and asked her to marry me. She said, "Yes!" So, you see ... nothing that has ever happened to me has stopped me from moving forward and living my best life. I believe that has EVERYTHING to do with my newfound relationship with God, THE ONE who, on my worst day, never left my side. He never abandoned me—and He never will.

# MEET CHRISTOPHER HOYER

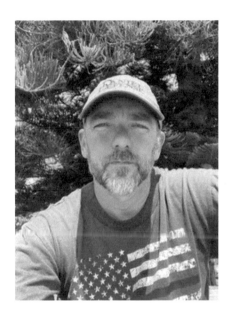

Retired Phoenix Police Officer, Christopher Hoyer, is a protector, survivor, and advocate for mental, physical, emotional, and spiritual wellness. After 20+ years as a street cop, having been faced with the worst horrors imaginable, he has turned his focus to sharing his story with others, helping the First Responder community prepare for the trauma that comes with the job. He has spoken to thousands, including First Responders, mental health professionals, and various professional entities, sharing his story in hope of saving lives. He is a professional speaker and the author of *When That Day Comes: Training for the Fight.*

~

## *Connect with Christopher*
### *Police Officer (Re.), Survivor, Advocate*

**Author of When That Day Comes: Training for the Fight**

*Email: Chrishoyer46@gmail.com*

~

# Your Turn

What came up for you in this story?

_____
_____
_____
_____
_____
_____
_____
_____
_____
_____
_____
_____
_____
_____
_____
_____
_____
_____
_____
_____
_____
_____
_____

# CHAPTER 23
# WHEN THE MASK CRACKED, EVERYTHING CHANGED

*By*
*Janet Wiszowaty*

Growing up, I never heard anyone talk about trauma, depression, or post-traumatic stress disorder (PTSD). It wasn't until I became a spouse of a police officer that I saw the effects of trauma. Still, I didn't understand what it was. What is not talked about or acknowledged is the fact that it affects everyone, from the person experiencing it to everyone around them.

In 2003, I was diagnosed with PTSD. As a spouse to a Royal Canadian Mounted police officer and a civilian member of the elite Canadian Police Force, I didn't realize there were traumatic events that led to my own diagnosis. It was never just one incident but an accumulation of incidents. Some were experienced as a spouse, comments made by my husband and his sudden change in behavior. He'd go from easygoing to short-tempered. That's when I found out about the calls he attended, involving the tragic death of children who were the same age as our children. He never talked about any of it with me; in 1975, that was how they trained.

When I joined the force and started working shiftwork and overtime, our marriage took on a new dynamic. With the shoe on the other foot, I understood a little more about him, and he began to understand more about me, too. Two specific incidents come to mind: 1.) When he was home alone, and I was at work, he would call to say it was lonely at home when I wasn't there, to which I would reply, "Welcome to My World!" 2.) I got home after midnight one shift because we were waiting on some urgent information. His first words to me were, "Did you put in for overtime?"

I put my hands on my hips and said the same thing he had said to me for ten years when he stayed past his scheduled shift, "Voluntary overtime!"

AFTER I STARTED DISPATCHING AND COMPLAINT TAKING, LOOKING after our members on the road, I never thought of being affected by the calls I took or the files we worked on. We just took each call and went on to the next one. The first time I realized it was affecting me was when a friend, a police officer, died by suicide. Dennis had attended a murder-suicide involving a child. He shared how he was having trouble rationalizing the event in his head. Six months later, he took his own life. In sharing his struggle, Dennis gave me a gift. I was better able to understand the earlier suicide of a family friend named Henry, the man who introduced me to my husband, Les. Henry died by suicide three days before our wedding, in the home of my future mother-in-law, and his funeral was on the same day as our wedding.

Over the years, I dealt with countless emergency calls and the deaths of other members I worked with; some were killed in the line of duty while others died by suicide. The calls that had an immediate impact on me were those involving children. As a mother, I felt helpless, as I had to remain calm and get help to them. It wasn't for many years that I would recognize the toll it took on my body. In 1991, I was diagnosed with fibromyalgia. My body was suffering from all that I could not consciously deal with. It was the equivalent of the old analogy of putting a frog into a pot of tepid water and then slowly turning up the temperature of the stove top. The frog, not registering any danger, wouldn't realize that he was boiling to death.

It took four motor vehicle accidents in ten years, each with a new injury, until the last one in August 2002 took me out for a whole year. All but the last accident caused physical injuries that I was able to work through with help. The last one was different because my mind was involved. The physical injuries would not allow me to do anything but sit and think. My life had been about raising kids, juggling activities, and shift work. It was easy to keep all the emotions stuffed down. There was no time to deal with them. That is when the mask cracked, and I had no control over what came up.

One night I found myself sitting in our living room—in the dark. Everyone in the house was asleep. I sat in my chair, silently crying, wishing I had died in that car accident. The mask I had been wearing for so long, the facade that helped me do my job as a police dispatcher, had cracked and all those suppressed emotions were coming up all at once.

Thankfully, I recognized that I needed help, and so I sought it. When my first psychologist was not a good fit, I went looking for another. Words of advice: Never work with someone you are not comfortable with. Fortunately, I found a good match. I honestly thought everything that was happening to me was because of the vehicle accidents. That turned out not to be the case. My psychologist diagnosed me with PTSD. She said, "What you are going through has everything to do with your job."

During my sessions, I developed tools to help me recover. While I still could not do much because of my physical injuries, I did a lot of reading. Books can be very healing. One of the books I read changed my life: *The Magic of Thinking Big* by David Schwartz. In the book, two men were conversing. One man (a clerk) was telling another man how he wanted to be a manager, but he was too busy listing all the reasons why he could not go back to school or start working toward becoming a manager. The other man looked at the clerk and, in so many words, told him that he had heard all the reasons why he *couldn't* become a manager and that he wanted him to go home and look for ways that he *could* become a manager. The man asked the clerk to come back in two weeks and share that new list.

*That simple analogy shifted my thinking.*

The accident in 2002 was the fourth I had been involved in within ten years. I like to believe that because I was not heading in the right direction after the first three, God made sure I was immobilized long enough for me to listen and learn. My knowledge grew from the books I read. It took a long time and a multitude of treatments, but I was finally mobile and able to go back to work. I was also able to carry two or three university courses per semester while working full-time.

I now count the accident as a blessing because doctors found some medical issues that had not yet made themselves known, and I was able to deal with them. In fact, the accident probably saved my life. Sometimes it takes being hit hard to wake us up. I learned that I was much stronger and smarter than I thought. I learned to live in and enjoy the present because it only takes a moment to lose everything. Life is for living. The past is behind me, and the present is a gift.

*My Five Stages Through PTSD:*

1) **Trauma**: Everyone experiences trauma sometime in their life. It may even go unacknowledged. For instance, until Dennis' suicide, I was not aware how much Henry's suicide had affected me.

2) **Awareness**: Until we can acknowledge that we have been living with unresolved trauma, we are unable to heal. It took multiple car accidents to raise awareness of what that unresolved trauma was doing to my mind and my body.

3) **Connection**: Until we acknowledge we need help, we are unable to connect with the right people to help us move through to recovery. I had a great psychologist, though she was not the only one to help me. I also worked with traditional medicine and non-traditional healers to get me to the next stage.

4) **Recovery**: Recovery is a journey. Although I was diagnosed over twenty years ago, there are still times that I get triggered. The goal is to keep moving forward. I continue to take courses, workshops, and surround myself with people who are willing to walk with me and support me on my journey. The Power of Our Story and the tribe Sara Correll brought together has been a huge thrust in my forward motion.

5) **Celebration**: I think celebration is a huge missing piece in the recovery process. I turned fifty the year I was diagnosed with PTSD. That September, I asked my daughter to plan a big birthday party for me. I needed to celebrate my 50th year with family and friends, while I was still around to enjoy it!

# MEET JANET WISZOWATY

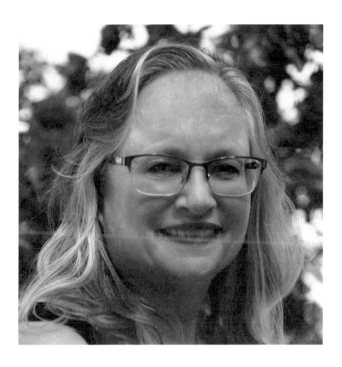

*"Life is a team sport, and when we all work together, miracles happen."*

In 1982, Janet Wiszowaty joined the Royal Canadian Mounted Police, a career spanning more than three decades. Following her husband, who was an RCMP officer, she worked in three Canadian Provinces and then went on to do relief work in two of Canada's three territories.

In 2003, she was diagnosed with Post Traumatic Stress

Disorder, resulting from a career working in the Operational Communications Centre as a police dispatcher and complaint taker. Since the diagnosis, Janet has made it her mission to transcend the trauma through therapy and education. She has found that by sharing her story and facilitating workshops and group sessions, she not only continues to move forward but is able to share tools with those she works with so that they are able to support themselves.

Janet is the chief connektor of Worldly ConneKtions, a life coach, a certified Canfield Success Principles trainer, a published author (*The Year the World Paused: Stories of Inspiration and Transformation*), and an international speaker who shared her story at the United Nations in 2017—the video is available on YouTube.

$\approx$

### Connect with Janet
**Royal Canadian Mounted Police/Dispatcher (Ret.)**

*Email: hello@janetwiszowaty.com*
*LinkedIn: Janet Wiszowaty*

$\approx$

# Your Turn

What came up for you in this story?

_____
_____
_____
_____
_____
_____
_____
_____
_____
_____
_____
_____
_____
_____
_____
_____
_____
_____
_____
_____
_____
_____
_____

# CHAPTER 24
# THE FIRE SERVICE: THE TEST OF ONE MAN'S METTLE

*By*

*Jim Lydon*

My career was filled with great experiences and memories of serving and helping others in the communities where I worked. This service was not just provided to the citizens but also to those with whom I worked. Although I am often reminded of these positive elements, I am also reminded of the impacts many events and circumstances had on my well-being.

My exposure to trauma began as an Explorer Scout at the age of fourteen. Impactful events included a suicide, a self-inflicted gunshot to the head, and a fire-related fatality. A teenager is not equipped for such experiences. From there, I started my career as a dispatcher at sixteen years old, progressing through the ranks of that organization for thirty-two years. The last six years were spent as a battalion chief.

Throughout my career, I experienced a lot of loss, including the loss of co-workers from illnesses and debilitating injuries. Some nearly lost their lives in the line of duty. I worked with some who suffered silently. Like me, they were dealing with the emotional toll of our profession. I watched as some destroyed themselves through substance abuse or other unhealthy coping mechanisms. And then, on the other side, there was the loss of innocent children and adults, people whose lives were tragically altered because of others' negligent actions. Working in the community where I grew up, I experienced incidents involving family, friends, and people I knew. Fortunately, I missed the call my crew took when my father suffered his final cardiac arrest. I likely would have been directly involved had I not been on leave. I was also at the center of several high-profile incidents where bureaucratic systems challenged the actions of me and/or my team.

On top of everything, I experienced personal challenges, like the emotional rollercoaster of finding out there was the potential for a significant health issue with our unborn child, only to find out we would be celebrating twins instead. And there was the loss of vision in one eye and the fear it would end my career. Despite it all, I continued in the profession for many years.

The emotional effects of traumatic events, especially early on in my career, led to coping mechanisms that were not the most appropriate. I would joke that I dealt with my emotions with a six-pack of beer in a dark room, listening to country music. That was my reality! I was relying on substances or other behaviors that weren't healthy or didn't promote solutions in the same way counseling or peer support do. However, this was common practice. I observed others in the profession doing the same. Later in my career, I understood the value of the more appropriate options and would advocate for support programs in the profession.

I left my original agency to become a fire chief in a nearby community, where I served in various positions at the City Manager's Office. Being selected for senior leadership brought many rewards over the years. One of the highlights was being able to launch someone's career or appoint them to a promoted position. The excitement they emitted when offered a position evoked an incredible feeling deep within me. On the opposite end of the spectrum was the complicated, sometimes emotionally draining decision to release someone from their position.

In some cases, this was due to their inability to meet standards. In other cases, it was due to the actions of the individuals. In either case, these were human beings, and my leadership decisions impacted their lives. Knowing this impacted my life. Often, I had a personal bond with these people during our service together. I also had to make decisions that affected the organization, or the service provided to the community. You will only ever understand the personal impact it has on you if you are in a position to make similar critical decisions. In many cases, rumors are started by individuals who are misinformed and unaware of all the details associated with the decision, which makes the situation even worse. It all has an impact on a leader's well-being.

As my career was winding down, I began pursuing the option to become assistant city manager and drop my role as fire chief. However, an opportunity arose that aligned with my future retirement plans, so I chose that path instead and became fire chief in yet another community. In my final days, before I switched organizations, I was involved in a difficult decision to terminate a peer. This included being present with him and assisting him for a few hours while he cleared out his personal belongings. Beyond dealing with the emotions of that process, I received a voicemail from one of his associates, threatening personal harm. I found comments on a community blog attacking me for my actions over the years as fire chief. These contributed to the emotional toll of my career.

It's not often a single event that compromises our mental well-being but rather the compounding effect of many events. For years, I got through challenges by having a good understanding of my purpose in life and the passion I had for achieving that purpose. Before I transitioned from the fire service, I was physically and emotionally drained. I was dealing with health issues and the impact of my leadership during the COVID-19 Pandemic. I was dealing with challenging personnel issues and suffering from the effects of these events. On top of all that, I was being asked to do things that did not align with my values, and the betrayal I was experiencing had taken its toll. I had been so focused on doing what I believed was right. I realized I could no longer achieve my purpose because my passion for the work I once enjoyed had waned. It was time to make a change. It all came to a head, and I said, "I am done."

Two weeks later, I began the next chapter of my life. Before the end of my fire service journey, job-related cancer and cardiac-related issues came into play, and I would continue to navigate those during my retirement. I put my heart and soul into this profession. I sacrificed myself and my family, only for the organization to dispute the job-related illnesses and attempt to attribute the impacts to other activities in my life. I got angry, which didn't help my health and well-being. Honestly, it even prevented me from being the person my family deserved. The dispute with my organization kept me from remaining focused on my life's purpose. All in all, I know that I experienced tremendous traumatic growth throughout my career. It has positioned me to be effective in what I do today, supporting those still serving their organizations and communities.

Two key components allowed me to overcome many of the challenges I experienced—professionally and personally. The first was the influence of my parents and the resiliency they modeled throughout their lives. They faced several personal challenges. However, they always seemed focused on overcoming adversity and moving forward. This modeled behavior allowed me to look past my challenges and focus on the future. For instance, when I lost sight in my eye, my original outlook was optimistic. I thought it would be okay because I had other skills and opportunities to tap into. Little did I know, I would not need to tap into those because remaining with the fire service was the best option.

The second component that helped me address challenges was "my circle," people I could count on for input and guidance. As I moved to various organizational roles, I found that my circle refined, based on my need to speak confidentially or open up to those at similar organizational levels. When I reached the position of fire chief and my roles within the City Manager's Office, I found my circle no longer existed—organizationally. I was reliant on those outside the organization. I recommend establishing a support network, including those outside your agency. Develop your circle so you can always "call a friend" when needed.

Although I had challenges throughout my journey, I was able to overcome them and remain focused on helping others adapt and rise above. Six months after retirement, I realized the importance of sharing my story. I go deeper each time I explore and reflect upon how I got here. I encourage you to take opportunities to explore and share your stories. Sharing your story with others helps to resolve existing negative impacts on your well-being. It enables you to understand the obstacles in your life better and how to get around them in a healthy way. I encourage you to live a life of purpose and make the necessary changes to avoid burnout. You deserve a successful career and the opportunity to walk out that door when the time comes as a physically and mentally healthy person.

# MEET JIM LYDON

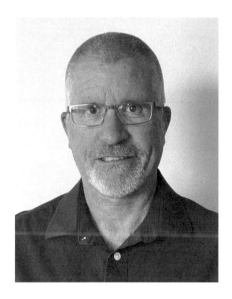

Jim Lydon spent 40 years in public service. His primary role was in the fire service, rising through the ranks to the position of fire chief in a city located in Northern California. He then had the opportunity to serve in the city manager's office as both an assistant city manager and city manager. Jim returned to the role of fire chief in a fire department in Southern California, where he finished his public service career. He now resides in San Diego with his wife and continues to serve, helping others grow as leaders through facilitation of a leadership development program, as well as personal coaching.

～

## *Connect with Jim*
*Public Servant, Fire Chief (Ret.), Leadership Development and Coaching*

*Email: lydonjal@gmail.com*
*LinkedIn: Jim Lydon*

～

# Your Turn

What came up for you in this story?

_____

_____

_____

_____

_____

_____

_____

_____

_____

_____

_____

_____

_____

_____

_____

_____

_____

_____

_____

_____

_____

_____

_____

_____

# CHAPTER 25
# EARN YOUR BADGE
# EVERY DAY

*By*
*David Berez*

It was 1989, and I was fourteen years old. I wanted to grow up to be a doctor, so I took the opportunity to join the volunteer rescue squad and begin, what I believed, would be my career in medicine. By sixteen years old, I earned my EMT certification along with many other secondary rescue certificates. At eighteen years old, I was certified as a heavy rescue technician, pre-hospital, trauma, life-support provider and several other specialties. I was well on my way to achieving my goal.

As a teenager, I was exposed to horrific car crashes, burn victims, drownings, infants I could not save, gunshot wounds, suicides, and homicides. As my EMS experiences mounted, along with my overall exposure to emergency services, I retooled my professional goals and decided that I wanted to become a police officer—a noble career where you get to help others, serve and engage your community, receive specialized training, and be part of a revered fraternity. Not to mention, the pay for police officers in New Jersey is about three times that of EMS.

In college, I tested the waters of law enforcement while working for the university's public safety department. I participated in two internships—the Freeport Police Department (NY), where I was introduced to the worst of humanity when I helped investigate the murder of an infant child who died at the hands of a parent and the East Windsor Police Department (NJ), where I spent my career. During my college years, I continued to volunteer as an EMT back home in East Windsor and on Long Island with the Uniondale Fire Department. I was exposed to many different calls for service and rescue missions, up to and including a passenger plane crash. It was also during my college tenure that I was faced with suicide for the first time—one of my mentors, a detective sergeant who worked in East Windsor. He became the subject of my senior thesis—*Critical Incident Stress Management*. I earned a dual degree in sociology and criminal justice.

Upon graduation from college, I had the good fortune of spending one year as a medicolegal intern with the New York City Medical Examiner's Office. There, I would assist with any and all death investigations that occurred in Manhattan. From unattended deaths of the elderly to mob hits; from "floaters" to rooftop jumpers, arson victims (crispy critters), and beyond. I literally had seen it all. The investigations included both on-scene and autopsies. To this day, I can still see and smell some of those cases.

I then went on to graduate the police academy in 1999 and begin my professional career as a police officer. A lot of interesting experiences occurred early on that gave shape to what path my career would take, but everything would change on September 11, 2001. I was off that day, but upon learning the news, I immediately headed into work where I met my partner—gear bags ready for deployment. Our agency made it clear that they were not going to send anyone because (and I quote) "Not our town; not our problem." With a bewildered look on our faces, my partner and I hopped into my personal car and drove up to Jersey City. There, we boarded a fire boat that took us to lower Manhattan.

We engaged in any way that we could and served to the best of our ability. While my time at Ground Zero remains as fuzzy as the pictures I took that day, the sights, the smells, the sounds, and the feelings are crystal clear. The experience shaped who I would become as an adult and as a police officer. I learned perspective. I learned priorities. I learned friendship and brotherhood. What I didn't know, is how long I would live with the nightmares.

As my career marched on, I was fortunate to have played many roles, had many experiences, and networked with many people. The good times and the positive impact I made on people and the community are too many to count and recall. They gave me great joy and pride, and it was truly an honor to have been part of them all. However, it is the moments of tragedy and loss that have impacted me the most—the car crash on an icy road where the driver, a father of three, hit another car head on, killing two of his three children. That man's shrills of despair are sounds I will hear to my own dying day. The death notification and the squeal of a mother's voice and emptiness in her eyes as I explained that her son died by suicide. Then, when she asked to see his body one last time, for one last hug, I had to explain to her that would not be possible since he jumped in front of a train. I will never forget holding a ten-year-old child in my arms as my partners unsuccessfully performed CPR on the only parent he had and then being the one to tell him he was now an orphan. To this day, I relive the time when I had to revive a childhood friend in the bathroom of a bar who still had the needle hanging from his arm which was the vehicle for the overdose. I still see the mangled body of another childhood friend with a Broadway career in her future, broadsided by an 18-wheeler.

I can still **see** the battered women, the abused children, the suicide hanging from the tree, the day laborer who fell into the commercial woodchipper on a rainy day. I **hear** the screams of a heartbroken parent, the screeching tires of my own car crashes, the loudest gun blast followed by deafening silence. I **smell** burning flesh, a rotting corpse, accelerants from fires, the ashes of a struggling man's business, the odor of alcohol on the breath of a soccer mom sitting behind the wheel of her minivan with a crushed front end, having just killed someone else's child. I can still **taste** the dust from the two fallen towers. But the fifth sense, **touch**, is the one I am challenged by the most. While my body aches from years of carrying the physical and emotional weight of the job and life experiences, it is the lack of touch where I endure the most pain. I can no longer feel my mother's embrace. I struggle to hug my own kids, and I am challenged by the inability to show affection to my wife because through it all, I have lost the ability to feel love.

I spent thirty years proudly serving my community in different capacities and stood tall through it all. I had collected a hundred lifetimes' worth of experiences and believed that each would make me stronger for the next. However, what I did not learn along the way would shape the second half of my life more than all I had learned. I did not know that these memories would be stored in a box that would eventually reopen, or should I say, explode open. I did not learn that each incident was a building block to an eventual post traumatic response. I did not understand that I would live with these events for the rest of my life.

After I retired in December of 2019, I still saw the look of sadness and despair, but only when I looked in the mirror. I still smelled the odor of alcohol, but it was on my own breath. I still heard a parent's desperate cry, but it stopped when I woke up from the nightmares. As I battle through thirty years' worth of memories, I find peace when I see the light in my children's eyes and the comfort in their hearts every morning when I wake them up and every night when I tuck them in. I feel the relief from my wife; she no longer worries when or if I'm coming home. I sense my own strength, both physical and mental, when I return from a fifty-mile bike ride, successfully working through a new challenge or achieving a new goal.

Following the suicidal death of a good friend and member of my Blue family, I realized something; not only was I not alone in my emotions, but I was in a much better place than many. My friend struggled with betrayal on many levels—from work to home, bosses to community and even the betrayal of his own mental health. Following his death, I experienced a feeling of guilt I had never felt before. As I worked to resolve my own pain, I found relief in helping others. I started by writing an article that reached over 15,000 people before being published nationwide. I then connected with another retired colleague who was the chief resilience officer for the county where I worked and lived. This resiliency program was what I needed for my own health and the ability to help others.

The resiliency program opened my mind. I learned to "count my blessings," "accomplish goals," "check my playbook," "balance my thinking," "capitalize my strengths," and utilize "acceptance strategies for mindfulness." As I apply these lessons and include physical and spiritual resilience, I strive to live more, love stronger, play harder, and find inner peace. While I work daily on a better me, I find the sweet spot in life is to help others find their best selves too.

If you are lost and struggling, find someone who can help light your path. If your path is well lit, find someone with whom you can share your light. In our Blue family, no one fights alone. Stay resilient and live a life full of purpose. This world is better because you are in it!

Life is a series of chapters, and when one comes to an end it is important to find a way and write the next so your story can continue. I found a new love of education that would reinforce the foundation of my purpose to serve others. Some may need to rebuild after their time in uniform and others may be able to build upon the success they earned in uniform. No matter your path, identify your purpose, fuel it, and live it in a new way that serves you best. There is life beyond the badge.

# MEET DAVID BEREZ

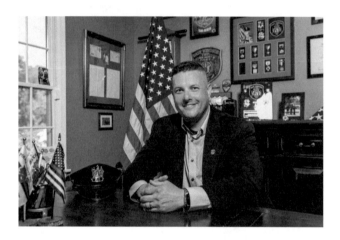

David Berez, a retired Police Officer and Drug Recognition Expert, served more than 20 years with the East Windsor Police Department and a total of 33 years in Emergency Services, including EMS and OEM. Following his retirement, Berez is now the president and founder of Six4 Consultants, a public safety consulting firm. He is the author of *A Resilient Life: A Cops Journey in Pursuit of Purpose*, a featured columnist, guest speaker, and panelist on a variety of public safety discussions. In September of 2020, Berez trained as a resiliency program officer and master resiliency trainer. He is a facilitator for Resilient Minds on the Front Lines, The Power of our Story, and is working to grow Resiliency for Law Enforcement Retirees in New Jersey with the state's Resilience Program. In 2022, Berez was named to the Law

Enforcement Advisory Counsel for Citizens Behind the Badge. He earned his Master of Applied Positive Psychology (MAPP) from the University of Pennsylvania, the foundational program in positive psychology. Berez is the first and only police officer to be accepted into this program and hold this degree. He completed his education with a capstone project focusing on emotional regulation in law enforcement officers through the use of the humanities. He believes that storytelling through literature and visual art can increase the wellbeing of the individual, communities, and institutions. Berez is now a positive psychology practitioner who teaches the use of positive interventions to support individuals, communities, and institutions to go beyond surviving and start thriving.

~

### Connect with David
#### MAPP, DRE

*Lead By Example. Stay Resilient. Earn Your Badge Every Day!*

*Author of A Resilient Life: A Cop's Journey in Pursuit of Purpose*

*Email: David@six4consultants.com*
*Website: www.Six4consultants.com*

~

# Your Turn

What came up for you in this story?

_____
_____
_____
_____
_____
_____
_____
_____
_____
_____
_____
_____
_____
_____
_____
_____
_____
_____
_____
_____
_____
_____
_____
_____
_____
_____
_____
_____

# CHAPTER 26
# GRIT, GRATITUDE, AND GRACE

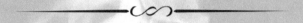

*by Michael S. DeSelm*

Shockwaves of searing pain pulsed throughout my body. As I lay underneath the Jeep on the rough asphalt, I didn't understand why … why this pain, why so intense, and why now. Fists clenched, tears welling up, I braced myself for the coming pain as I got to my feet. Gingerly making my way into the house, another wave of pain coursed through my body, bringing me to my knees. I collapsed onto the carpeted floor. Hunched over the ottoman, my son looked at me quizzically, almost as confused and helpless as me.

For months, I could tell that something in my body wasn't "right." Running became painful, workouts hurt, and recovery took forever. I was confident that I'd pulled a muscle in my back or, worse, herniated a disc. I got new shoes, started doing yoga, and focused on working my core, all with minimal relief.

Nevertheless, I'd walk the dog every day and try to keep to the routines that kept my mental health in check. What had started as a dull ache in my hips and lower back progressed to a severe limp and near-intractable pain.

Leery of doctors with sharp objects, I sought answers through chiropractic functional medicine that included three weekly adjustments, handfuls of supplements, focused stretching, and even massage therapy. You'd think after three months, a reprieve would come, but it didn't; the pain just kept getting worse. Reluctantly, I went to the doctor. Like me, the doctor agreed that my symptoms were reasonably consistent with a herniated disc and ordered an MRI to confirm. While the idea of climbing into a loud, clanging torpedo-tubed imaging machine did not excite me, I needed answers, so I could stop this pain that had taken over my life.

I spent fourteen-plus years in the Navy as a Hospital Corpsman, serving in a multitude of roles. After nearly seven years working in hospitals, I grew restless and wanted something more than standing around an OR, passing instruments (and my life) away ... so I went to dive school in the summer of 2002 to become a Diving Medical Technician. Though I graduated as the class honor man, I was skittish in the water column. I never admitted it then, but I'm a bit claustrophobic and maybe a little high-strung. It still blows my mind that I even made it through. I went on to have a successful tour that lasted six-and-a-half years at SDVT-2 in Little Creek, Virginia. Perhaps it was a little more than ironic; submarines were our primary platform. I am still baffled that I survived all those sub-trips. How anyone can trust a nineteen-year-old, pimple-faced noob with a PlayStation controller to drive a multibillion-dollar nuclear submarine in the dark waters of the ocean is beyond me. The thought of dying trapped in a submarine doesn't seem like an unreasonable fear to me.

"Heterogeneous abnormal marrow signal in the L1 and L3 vertebral body" is what the report said. As I sat on the beach, watching my kids splash in the waves, my mind raced. How was I going to explain to them the road that lay before me, before us as a family, that cancer had invaded my body and its outcome uncertain? My phone rang. It was the doctor.

"Michael, you have to come into the hospital immediately," he said. "Your MRI results are in, and we need to run more tests." I cut him off, having already read the report on my phone. "Doc, I've been in pain for months. I'm sitting on a beach right now, enjoying the day with my family. Your tests can wait until I come back next week on Monday." I was not going to allow him, or the previously undiagnosed cancer eating away at my hip and spine, to rob me of this moment with those most precious to me. Besides, this only confirmed what we all feared to be true, unspoken until now.

There is something to be said about one's ability to endure adversity. Life is filled with moments that will test your mettle, challenge your thinking, and allow you to dig deep. While many words describe these moments, I gravitate to the word *grit*; it has substance. You can feel it when you say it: *grit*. One of my favorite shirts from Dive School had the phrase *"illegitimi non carborundum"* inscribed across the back. Loosely translated, it means don't let the bastards grind you down, a fitting ode to *grit*. It had taken *grit* to get this far; it would take more to navigate the road ahead.

"Yup, it's what we expected," the oncologist said. I'd just

recently completed a biopsy and then a PET Scan to diagnose and evaluate what kind of beast we were fighting. "Non-Hodgkin's Lymphoma. Now, it's Stage IV due to bone marrow involvement, but our treatment plan is curative."

The PET scan showed that I had cancer in my lumbar spine, the right iliac crest of my pelvis, my right hip, and all the lymph nodes in between. I even had some in my ribs, but thankfully, no central organ involvement. As I hung up the phone, my teenage son looked at me and asked, "When you lose all your hair, can I put a plunger on your head?" Laughing, I scowled at him and told him to bugger off. Looking back, I'm thankful for my family's use of sarcasm to bring levity to uncomfortable situations. For the next five months, I lived my life twenty-one days at a time. Never looking too far ahead, my singular focus was to survive the current round of chemo and get to the next round, twenty-one days later.

Nothing quite prepares you for the marathon that is chemotherapy. They tell you what will happen, but it never seems "real" until the moment it becomes so. As expected, and much to my son's chagrin, I lost all my hair. Thankfully, my head is just a bit too round to support his plunger idea. What I didn't expect was how much I would miss my eyelashes and how they protect your eyes (I endured multiple eye infections throughout treatment). I was not prepared for the weight *gain*. I easily gained at least thirty pounds throughout treatment. I remember thinking, "Jeez, God, I thought I was signing up for the weight loss program!"

Worst of all, I was not prepared for the "I'm stranded alone on a desert island" feeling of isolation that cancer created—like I was utterly and totally alone. The COVID pandemic had forced a level of isolation on all of us already; cancer doubled down on that.

I am incredibly thankful to have built a strong local support network beyond my amazing wife and kids. I owe a debt of *gratitude* to three dear friends who met with me on Zoom most every morning—a practice we had begun due to COVID. Aside from near-daily check-ins, what I valued most about these men was that they never treated me like a cancer patient. I was their brother in arms, someone of value, with perspective to give and a heart to serve. They reminded me to be fully present in every moment—be it pain or joy, as every moment is something to be *grateful* for. My life is richer because of their investment in me. I still meet with these guys today, seeking to impart wisdom and perspective, praying that I might support them when their time of grit comes to bear.

In retrospect, I've become more aware of the impact, importance, and value of *grace*. Call it unmerited favor or, to honor and give credit to, *grace* simply put, is a gift you didn't earn. To live is *grace*. Every moment is precious; every second is worth a lifetime. None of us knows what today might bring; tomorrow is promised to no one. But today ,,, today, you have a choice. Get up, get out, and grind … or wallow in the depths of your circumstances. The choice is yours, and you have to fight for it. Look inward; look outward; look upward. Find something worth fighting for and grab it with all your conviction. Find a few good friends who will walk with you through the slog. You already know who they are; they are waiting for you to invite them into your fight. They are as grateful for you as you are for them. And, when all is said and done, be kind to yourself. Do what you can today to laugh a little longer, love a little deeper, and make sure those in your sphere of influence know how much you value them.

〜

You've got *grit*—you can make it if you are willing to grind.
Embrace *gratitude*—be fully present in every moment.
Go live in the *grace* afforded you today.

# MEET MICHAEL DESELM

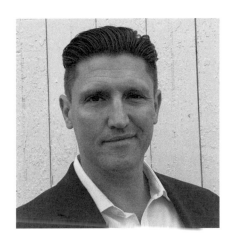

Not big on titles or accolades, Michael DeSelm's story is no different than so many others--he's just a dude who abides and wants the best for people. He's had adversity to overcome, heartbreak to endure, loss to survive, and hurt to make amends for. He found success after failure and battled the inner voices of imposter syndrome while serving with some of this nation's most dedicated and decorated professionals. He is a husband, a father, a brother, a Veteran, and a cancer survivor. Ultimately, though, he is just a dude who is thankful for today, looking to be fully present in every moment. Michael is the senior manager of Corporate Partnerships at Stop Soldier Suicide; he seeks to build and expand relationships with organizations, connecting their philanthropic interests to support Veteran and Service Members' mental health.

∾

### *Connect with Michael*
**USN Veteran, Dive Med Tech, Cancer Survivor, Veteran Advocate**

*Email: Michael.deselm@gmail.com*
*LinkedIn: Michael DeSelm, MBA*
*Website: www.padremikeyd.com*

∾

# Your Turn

What came up for you in this story?

_____

_____

_____

_____

_____

_____

_____

_____

_____

_____

_____

_____

_____

_____

_____

_____

_____

_____

_____

_____

_____

_____

_____

_____

_____

# CHAPTER 27
# EMBRACING CRISIS: A JOURNEY OF GROWTH, RESILIENCE, AND FAITH

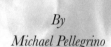

*By*
*Michael Pellegrino*

I n life, we encounter storms that test our resilience, challenge our beliefs, and shake the very foundations of our existence. For some, these storms may seem insurmountable, but for others, they become opportunities for growth and transformation. This is a story of navigating through the tumultuous waters of crisis, finding light in the darkness, and emerging stronger on the other side.

The journey began with my wife, Diana, and I facing a series of challenges that rocked our world. We had suffered multiple miscarriages and, ultimately, were unable to have children. While dealing with infertility, Diana's company decided to downsize, eliminating her high-paying position, leaving us both feeling lost and uncertain about the future. It was a time when it seemed like the world was conspiring against us, testing our faith and resilience in ways we could never imagine. In the midst of this storm, I turned to the skills of resilience I hadn't even cultivated yet.

Dealing with infertility while managing numerous responsibilities at work was incredibly challenging. For both my wife and I, the ache of not being parents was profound. Receiving the life-changing news was overwhelming, stirring up a mixture of thoughts and feelings, including sadness, frustration, and uncertainty about the future. Our strong marriage and love for each other helped us tremendously, as we navigated this difficult journey together.

I recall the struggles of working as a police officer—the unusual shifts and responding to calls while grappling with the possibility of Diana and I never having children. One vivid memory stands out. It was Thanksgiving night. While our family gathered for dinner downstairs, Diana was upstairs experiencing a miscarriage. Despite the heartbreaking situation, we didn't want to dampen anyone's spirits. So, I found myself going up and down the stairs, checking on everyone—first the family eating dinner downstairs and then making sure my wife was doing okay upstairs. It was a delicate balance between attending to family festivities and caring for Diana during a deeply challenging moment.

Gratitude has always been my lifeline. I focus on the blessings in my life rather than dwelling on what I lack. I find solace in the simple joys of everyday moments, recognizing the beauty in the present, despite the uncertainty that looms ahead. I know that as long as Diana and I have each other, we can face anything together.

Mindfulness plays a crucial role in my journey, too. I learned to quiet the noise of my racing thoughts and fears, finding peace in the stillness of my mind. Rather than being consumed by worry and anxiety, I embrace each moment with a sense of acceptance allowing myself to be fully present in the here and now.

But perhaps the most transformative aspect of my journey is in finding purpose and meaning amidst the chaos. In the face of adversity, I turn inward, seeking guidance and strength from my faith in God. It is through prayer and reflection that I discovered a sense of purpose beyond my own struggles—a higher calling that gave meaning to my experiences and inspired me to persevere.

As I navigate through life's storms, I realize that resilience isn't just about bouncing back from adversity; it is about forging new pathways in the brain, rewiring my thoughts and beliefs to find hope and optimism in the face of despair. Through perseverance and determination, I have begun to see the silver linings hidden within the clouds, embracing the challenges as opportunities for growth and self-discovery.

Diana and I embarked on an entrepreneurial journey that began with a shared vision: to establish an advertising and marketing company specializing in digital billboards. As we delved into this venture, we encountered challenges and opportunities that would shape our trajectory in unforeseen ways. The dynamic landscape of the digital marketing industry demanded adaptability and innovation, qualities we were determined to embody.

One pivotal aspect of our journey was learning how to navigate the realm of real estate acquisitions to expand our company's portfolio. This presented us with a unique set of challenges, from understanding market trends to negotiating deals and managing properties. Through diligent research, networking, and seeking guidance from seasoned professionals, we honed our skills and gradually built a diverse real estate portfolio. Each acquisition not only bolstered our company's assets but also provided valuable insights into the intricacies of property management and investment strategies. However, our aspirations extended beyond business success; we sought to make a meaningful impact in the community and pursue our passion for mental wellness advocacy. This led us to establish Resilient Minds On The Front Lines, a platform dedicated to promoting mental wellness and resilience, particularly among frontline workers. Drawing from our personal experiences and insights gained from our professional endeavors, we envisioned a space where individuals could access resources, support, and guidance to navigate the challenges of their respective fields while prioritizing their mental well-being.

I retired as a police officer in 2019. When COVID hit, I was working for the Mercer County Prosecutor's Office as the chief resiliency officer. As we launched the webcast series "Resilient Minds on the Front Lines," we reached audiences in 76 countries and all 50 states. My wife and I realized we needed to do more, so we sold our house and moved into a garage apartment to finance our passion. We assembled a group of doctors and subject matter experts to develop the curriculum. After ten months and three pilot classes, we refined the program. We started as a nonprofit and have since expanded to a for-profit as well. We are constantly refining, improving, developing relationships, and living our purpose.

Central to the success of Resilient Minds On The Front Lines was the formation of our "Resilient Minds Family." Comprising subject matter experts and doctors in the field of mental health, this diverse group of individuals brought a wealth of knowledge, experience, and compassion to our initiative. Collaborating with them was not only enriching but also deeply inspiring. Their unwavering dedication to improving mental health outcomes resonated with our mission, propelling us forward with renewed purpose and determination.

The synergy within our Resilient Minds Family was palpable,

fostering an environment of mutual respect, empathy, and support. Each member contributed their unique perspectives and expertise, enriching our collective efforts to promote mental wellness. Together, we developed comprehensive programs, workshops, and resources tailored to the specific needs of not only frontline workers but EVERYONE, addressing topics such as stress management, resilience building, and coping strategies.

One of the most rewarding aspects of our journey was witnessing the transformative impact of our initiatives on individuals and communities. Through Resilient Minds On The Front Lines, we had the privilege of connecting with workers from various sectors, hearing their stories, and providing them with the tools and support they needed to thrive in challenging environments. Witnessing their resilience and determination in the face of adversity reaffirmed our belief in the power of this program and the collective action of each individual, whether they were a student or facilitator.

Throughout our journey, one sentiment echoed consistently —"It's NOT about me; it's about we." This profound realization underscored the importance of collaboration, teamwork, and shared purpose in achieving our goals.

Looking ahead, we are filled with excitement and optimism for the future. Our journey has been marked by growth, resilience, and meaningful connections, and we are committed to building upon these foundations to create a lasting impact. Whether it's expanding our business ventures, furthering our advocacy efforts, or nurturing our relationships within the Resilient Minds Family, Diana and I are driven by a shared vision of making a positive difference in the world. Our journey—from infertility to a job layoff to police work to founding an advertising and marketing company to establishing Resilient Minds On The Front Lines—has been a testament to the power of passion, perseverance, and collaboration. Through our experiences, we have learned valuable lessons, forged meaningful connections, and made a tangible impact in the lives of others. As we continue to chart our course forward, we do so with gratitude for the journey thus far and excitement for the adventures that lie ahead. It was our strong marriage and love for each other, matched with the collective effort of our team, partners, and community that fueled our significance and success to propel us forward.

～

*Be safe.*
*Be healthy.*
*Be resilient!*

～

# MEET MICHAEL PELLEGRINO

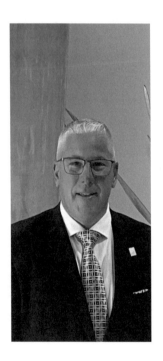

Michael Pellegrino, author of *Crisis = Opportunity*, certified motivational speaker, life coach, and real estate agent in New Jersey and Florida, has a distinguished career in law enforcement, education, and community service. After graduating from Notre Dame High School in Lawrenceville, New Jersey, he continued his education at Caldwell College and the Martin School of Business in Philadelphia, Pennsylvania.

Michael launched his law enforcement career at 19 years old, graduating from the Trenton Police Academy in 1994. He served on the Patrol Division, as well as various other roles, including traffic officer, and school resource officer, where he taught Drug Abuse Resistance Education (DARE) and Gang Resistance Education and Training (GREAT) programs. He worked closely with students, fostering strong community relations. As a detective for the Ewing Police Department, he showcased his commitment to public safety.

Michael's dedication earned him numerous accolades, such as the Ewing Police Medal of Honor, New Jersey State Policemen's Benevolence Association (PBA) Unit Citation Award, National Police Officer of the Month, and the Carnegie Medal of Honor. He served in leadership roles within the New Jersey State PBA, including 2nd Vice President. Retiring after 25 years, Michael became chief resiliency officer for Mercer County. He and his wife, Diana, own DPM Shore Solutions, an advertising and event company. Michael is the founder of Resilient Minds on the Front Lines, LLC, where creating and maintaining a resilient mindset begins.

≈

### Connect with Michael
**Detective (Ret.), Ewing Police Department (New Jersey)**

*Email: mpellegrino@resilientminds.us*
*Website: www.resilientminds.us*
*Website: www.crisisequalsopportunity.us*
*Crisis = Opportunity: Finding Growth and*
*Resilience in Challenging Times*

≈

# Your Turn

What came up for you in this story?

_____

_____

_____

_____

_____

_____

_____

_____

_____

_____

_____

_____

_____

_____

_____

_____

_____

_____

_____

_____

_____

_____

_____

_____

# CHAPTER 28
# YA GOTTA OWN YOUR CONDITION!

———∽———

*By*
*Gregg F. Martin*

## THE STORM

I received a call on a Friday afternoon in mid-July 2014. I was told to report to my boss, General Martin Dempsey, the Chairman of the Joint Chiefs of Staff (CJCS), on Monday morning at 10:00 a.m. The chairman also invited my wife, Maggie. In my sick brain, I wondered, "Will this be a promotion? An extension in command? Or will I be fired?"

I had worked for General Dempsey four times in my career. We had a great relationship. I reported to him as requested that day, and I saluted him. He strode across his office and gave me a big hug.

"Gregg, I love you like a brother," he said. "You've done an amazing job, a grade of A+. No one could have achieved what you've done, and in just two years, but your time at National Defense University is over. You have until 5:00 pm today to resign or you're fired! And I'm ordering you to get a psychiatric evaluation this week at Walter Reed."

*Do you think I was disappointed?*

*NO!*

"Thank you, Chairman!" I declared, hugging him. "God put me in this job. He removed me, and now He's got bigger things for me to do!"

That same month, I underwent three psychiatric evaluations, each while in a state of full-blown mania. And three times I was misdiagnosed as "fit for duty." Growing up, I had a hyperthymic personality. I was in a near-constant state of mild mania. Unknowingly living on the bipolar spectrum *helped me* for years with extra energy, drive, and enthusiasm. I excelled at key commands and military schools and in civilian grad school at MIT, where my mission was to obtain a master's degree in engineering. I came out with two master's degrees and a PhD.

*My bipolar brain at work!*

Hyperthymia enhanced my talents, but I was slowly inching my way up the spectrum toward bipolar disorder.

Throughout my career, as I was being promoted from colonel to one-star general, then to two-star general, my bipolar disorder was flying under the radar, unknown, unrecognized, and undiagnosed. Meanwhile, I cycled into higher highs and lower lows, with psychosis. I was a key commander in fierce combat, rapidly anticipating and creating solutions to complex, unexpected problems while under fire, often making near-simultaneous life-and-death decisions. This altered the wiring and chemistry of my brain. In 2003, I shot into my first mania when we attacked from Kuwait into Iraq. I felt like Superman and performed brilliantly, by all accounts. Upon redeployment to Germany, the thrill of combat behind me, I fell into a 10-month depression. That was my first full up-down bipolar disorder cycle. Bipolar disorder mostly helped me, until it didn't.

By 2014, I had skyrocketed into full-blown mania—madness and insanity. I was disruptive, bizarre, over-the-top, frightening, and out of control. I swung from euphoria to agitation, to anger, and to rage—infused with delusions, hallucinations, and extreme paranoia. I stopped sleeping for about three months. My speech became more rapid and pressured. New ideas flowed continuously. My grandiosity and religiosity soared. I talked nearly non-stop. I stopped doing paperwork. My meetings ran over, and I constantly interrupted conversations. I was repeatedly late, often out of uniform, and my risk-taking and lack of self-control were severe. I believed I could fly and that I was the smartest person on Earth. I believed I held the key to world peace and was God's apostle on a mission to transform the National Defense University (NDU) and Department of Defense (DOD). I saw the Holy Spirit descend and watched as demons attacked our house. I repelled them with Bibles and crosses … and much more. People noticed and began sending dozens of anonymous reports to my boss, leading to my removal from command.

## WHAT GOES UP, MUST COME DOWN

After being fired, I was retired early and later hospitalized. During these months, my psychotic brain convinced me that disgruntled employees had set me up for the fall and orchestrated my firing, and the three "fit for duty" psychiatric exams were proof of my fitness. My happy mania transformed into intense bitterness, anger, and rage. I felt betrayed by my people and the military I had served for 35 years, even though I realized General Dempsey had done me a huge favor that day by removing me from the snake pit and saving me from a possible stroke, heart attack, and/or the worst of my acute mania.

Over the next four months, I spiraled, then crashed into a

complete breakdown—mind, body, and spirit. I went from euphoric mania to hopelessness, crippling depression, and terrifying psychosis. I had never felt so weak, crippled, and helpless. As my sick brain caused me to descend into bipolar hell, things went from bad to worse over the next two years! It was indescribably awful, and I had NO HOPE! I believed I would NEVER recover!

*I wanted to die.*

In November 2014, I walked into Walter Reed and was *finally* diagnosed properly with bipolar disorder type I and psychotic features—twelve years after onset. Both the VA and the Army determined that my onset was in 2003, at the age of forty-seven, during the Iraq War and that my genetic predisposition for bipolar disorder was triggered by the stress, thrill, and euphoria of leading thousands of soldiers in combat.

I decided, right then and there, that I would OWN my diagnosis and that I would NOT be stigmatized, ashamed, or embarrassed. Those feelings are all based on fear and ignorance. Bipolar disorder is physiologically REAL, like diabetes, cancer, and heart disease, so I was not about to allow anyone to stigmatize me for my brain disease!

*And I haven't!*

I hugged and thanked my doctor, telling him that I finally had a target with a face on it—bipolar disorder type I and psychosis.

~

### FROM 2014 TO 2016, I LIVED IN BIPOLAR HELL

For two years, I was sunk in hopeless depression, barely functioning, and I kept getting worse! I had terrifying psychosis: delusions of being spied on, arrested, beaten, stabbed, and murdered in prison, face down, gurgling in a pool of my own blood. I had continuous ideations of my own death.

*I had a strong desire* to die!

I could feel a powerful, invisible force throwing me under a speeding 18-wheeler and steer me into on-coming trucks. Every morning, a giant boa constrictor slithering out of the woods, eyes blazing and tongue flickering, crushed the life out of me. These morbid thoughts of death and dying are called "passive suicidal ideations." In my mind and spirit, they were REAL. I could feel and smell my own death.

When I wasn't staring off into space and ruminating about every mistake I made in my life, I threw myself onto the hardwood floors, yelling, banging my head, and punching myself in the face and head. I was angry at God. Thankfully, my wonderful wife, Maggie, and a devoted friend and battle buddy got me into a great VA hospital for excellent inpatient care. A multi-disciplinary team of medical professionals treated and cared for me, lifting my spirits. The amazing VA chaplain helped me through with her compassionate, spiritual care. This treatment stabilized me and kept me from getting worse, but it was still six more months of bipolar hell, until lithium—a natural salt harvested from the earth—saved me.

∽

### AUGUST 2016: WITH LITHIUM, BEGAN MY JOURNEY OF *Recovery*

I say "journey" because I'm in a "forever war." There is no cure and no end to this. I must own and manage my bipolar disorder every day, for life. I started lithium in August 2016 and, within days, my symptoms miraculously vanished. I felt good and happy for the first time in years. My energy and interests returned.

*Medications are critical!*

My wife and I moved to Florida for the sunshine and warmth, and I began feeling like my old, pre-bipolar self.

*Place matters!*

It took a team to lift me up, including my wife, family, friends, medical professionals, and religious leaders. They gave me the hope and knowledge that I ***could and would*** recover.

*People are key!*

Bipolar disorder can strike anyone—young and old, rich and poor, educated and illiterate, privates and generals, male and female, all races. If left untreated, bipolar disorder often ruins marriages, families, careers, finances, and often leads to homelessness, addiction, prison, violence, and suicide. Today, my life is happy, healthy, and purposeful. I'm thriving! My hyperthymic personality is back, though less intense, and my bottom line is that there is HOPE! Recovery is possible. I am living proof! We've got to OWN our condition. If we don't, then it will own us! My life's mission is to share my story and to help stop the stigma, promote recovery, and save lives. It's a cause bigger than myself and it serves others. I LOVE it!

### MY STRATEGY FOR RECOVERY IS MULTI-DIMENSIONAL

Firstly, medications are for balancing my brain chemistry. I will take them every day, for life. These pills are my friends. ***I need them!*** Secondly, therapy is very important! Plus, keeping my wife Maggie close, wired in, and engaged as my battle buddy. Thirdly, I maintain healthful living—diet, sleep, exercise, water, low stress, etc. These first three strategies are necessary but not sufficient for a recovery that's built to last. They must be anchored into the 5P's:

1. **Purpose**: Find or create a life mission that drives you forward. [*]
2. **People**: Surround yourself with happy, fun, energetic people who lift you up. [†]
3. **Place**: Live where you want and where you can pursue your dreams. [‡]
4. **Perseverance**: Cultivate the will to win and never give up. [§]
5. **Perspective**: Develop the ability to get out of your own head and think objectively about your own thoughts, or metacognition.[#]

***Bottom line: Ya Gotta OWN Your Condition!***

---

[*] Dr Thomas Insel's *Healing: Our Path from Mental Illness to Mental Health*, Penguin Press, New York, 2022, see pp. 160-78, 239, 241.
[†] Dr Thomas Insel's *Healing: Our Path from Mental Illness to Mental Health*, Penguin Press, New York, 2022, see pp. 160-78, 239, 241.
[‡] Dr Thomas Insel's *Healing: Our Path from Mental Illness to Mental Health*, Penguin Press, New York, 2022, see pp. 160-78, 239, 241.
[§] https://www.psychiatrictimes.com/view/the-4-ps-of-mental-recovery-medical-care-and-healthfulness
[#] https://www.psychiatrictimes.com/view/the-4-ps-of-mental-recovery-medical-care-and-healthfulness

# MEET GREGG F. MARTIN

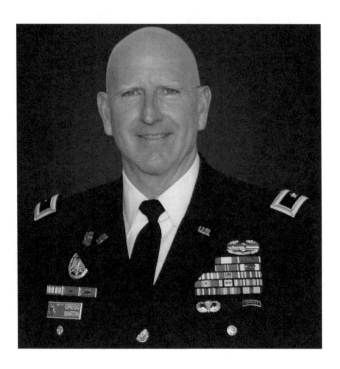

Major General Gregg F. Martin, Ph.D., US Army (Ret.), aka the BIPOLAR GENERAL, is a 36-year Army Combat Veteran, bipolar survivor, thriver, warrior, and a retired Two-Star General. He commanded an engineer company and battalion, as well as the 130th Engineer Brigade during the first year of the Iraq War. A former president of the National Defense University, commandant of the Army War College, and commander of Fort

Leonard Wood, Gregg is a qualified Airborne Ranger Engineer and strategist who holds a bachelor's degree, four master's, and a Ph.D. from West Point, MIT, and both the Army and Naval War colleges.

Gregg unknowingly lived most of his life on the bipolar spectrum, which largely enhanced his performance as a leader until it skyrocketed, ending his career, throwing him into crisis, leading to hospitalization, and nearly destroying him. Now, in his eighth year of bipolar recovery, he is an author, speaker, and ardent mental health advocate who lives with his wife in Cocoa Beach, Florida. He has three sons—two who live with bipolar disorder (an artist and a poet/Special Forces Veteran) and one who is an Army Special Forces Officer. Gregg's life's mission is to share his bipolar story to help stop the stigma, promote recovery, and save lives. His new book, *Bipolar General: My Forever War with Mental Illness*, is available on Amazon and is co-published by the Naval Institute Press (Jack Clancy's first publisher) and the Association of the US Army.

❧

### Connect with Gregg,
**Major General, US Army (Ret.)**

**Author of Bipolar General: My Forever War With Mental Illness**

*Website: www.bipolargeneral.com*

❧

# Your Turn

What came up for you in this story?

_____
_____
_____
_____
_____
_____
_____
_____
_____
_____
_____
_____
_____
_____
_____
_____
_____
_____
_____
_____
_____
_____
_____
_____
_____
_____
_____

# ACKNOWLEDGMENTS

———————⟨∽⟩———————

What a journey this has been and I could not have done it without my husband, Jon. Thank you for giving me the support to focus on creating a place of safety for those who have protected us. I'm so thankful for our sons, Connor, Hunter, Garrett and Wyatt, who taught me so much about love and connection through motherhood. I love you so much! I'm grateful for our wonderful daughters-in-law, Bekah and Lauren, and our grandbabies, Maverick and Parker Rae. What a gift you all are. To all our close friends, you have taught me so much through our friendships. You all are a big part of me wanting to pass the gift of tribe and community on to others, as I know personally the healing that comes from that.

What an honor it is to be surrounded by those who believe in serving something greater than themselves. It has been an extraordinary experience, and I thank you all for making me feel so at home with you!

To all our 29 Authors, you made this challenging journey of writing a book so sweet. I have such deep respect for every single one of you. You have put yourselves out there so deeply so that others can find their own voice and start the healing journey. Thank you for protecting our Protectors through your stories. 🙏 I am honored to call you my friends.

Where would we be without our group facilitators who have spent hours caring and leading talks on The Power Of Our

Story! Thank you, Michelle Collier (Franklin), Aaron Terrill and Sarah-Marie Baumgartner, Joel Landi, Jeremy Gronau, Barry Zworestine, Scott Duncan, Janet Wiszowaty, Dave Weiner, Christopher Gregorio, David Berez, Patrick McCurdy, Paul Curtis, "Chappie" Todd Stewart, Holly Higgins, Daniel Torrez, Jim Lydon, Paula Wold, and Anthony Ball. YOU have sustained our tribe with your heart for others and a deep desire to welcome all who are suffering in silence. You have given so many a home with us and it has been a joy to watch people gain their confidence back and thrive!! I'm so grateful for your friendship and collaboration. 🙏 There have been so many that have been with us along the way that we know are just a phone call away.

I want to thank others behind the scenes who have been such a big part of building this tribe of Protectors and supporting our book. A big THANK YOU to Michelle Collier (Franklin) who stepped up and volunteers her time to be our wonderful social media coordinator and friend. Thank you to Deny Caballero with Security Halt! Media, who generously produced our mini series for our book. Thank you to our editor, Natalie June Reilly, for genuinely having a heart for our Protectors and making sure their stories flow. Thank you to (Ret.) US Navy SEAL, Scott Rathke, who gave me the final push to facilitate and get this book written. Your input and belief means so much to me.

Thank you, John Walker, Co-Founder at Holo Sail Technologies Inc., for supporting our website since 2020. What a gift!

Thank you, Judith Richardson Schroeder, Chief Executive Officer - Publisher of Carnelian Moon Publishing Inc., who has been so kind and supportive through this whole process. Thank you to Tanja Prokop for your beautiful book cover design.

*Much love to you all,*
*Sara*

# ABOUT THE EDITOR

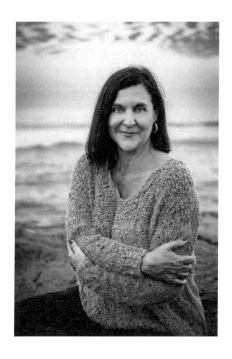

*Natalie June Reilly*

Over the past 25 years, I have been blessed with a prolific writing and editing career. It has not been without patience, persistence, extra thick skin, and God's grace. In the early days, I was a community columnist for the Arizona Republic. I have written scores of articles for magazines across the country, as well as internationally. I published *My Stick Family*, a children's book on divorce, the old-fashioned way, through a small publishing house out of New Jersey—49 rejections later. I wrote for the school paper in college—Arizona State University—Go Devils! At that same rag, I got my first taste of being an opinions editor. And I was good at it. Moreover, I loved it!

I've sold more than 15 stories to the Chicken Soup for the Soul series. I was commissioned to write two autobiographies—one for a former professional NBA player/self-made millionaire and one for a former US Marshal (who you'll hear from in this book). I've self-published two books of my own (*All Because of a Love Note* and *Pax the Polar Bear*) and edited and helped publish seven that have recently hit bookshelves ... with two on the way. Two of those authors are included in this book.

I can't help but feel that my writing career was always leading me to this project and to these people—my people. I, a former suburban, football mom who watches Christmas movies in July and who can't seem to open up a jar of pickles or peanut butter without help, know nothing of war or street violence or serious trauma, other than what I've seen in movies and read about in books. How would I know what it feels like to come home with the weight of *that* world on my shoulders? Yet, here I am, helping these courageous men and women share their stories, and I've never felt more at home.

What I lack in front-line experience, I make up for in love, gratitude, and the ability to listen. Listening, after all, is the key to effective communication. For a handful of years now, I have listened to some of my best friends who have served their country and communities tell stories of how they have been shot at, spit on, stabbed, ambushed, broken, betrayed, and wounded in ways that remain unseen to the human eye. They have been demonized by the media and oftentimes thrown to the wolves by their own agencies for reasons that cannot be explained, except to say they did not buckle under the pressures of the job and the powers that be. A few of them came close—too close for comfort. However, I am proud to say that they are still standing to this day. More importantly, they are *standing up* to tell their stories. Now, that takes real courage!

As the mother of a United States Navy Veteran/Texas law enforcement officer and the sweetheart and soon-to-be bride of a retired street cop, I have a profound respect for our Protectors. Seriously ... nothing but love! My dad served in the United States Army, and two of my great uncles, Martin and Gabriel Tafoya, served in World War II—both went missing in action during the Bataan Death March. The bodies of these two brothers from New Mexico were never recovered. They didn't make it home, and their mother was never the same. These young men who died for their country will never have the opportunity to share their stories, which is why the stories within these pages are so important to the fabric of our nation, not to mention surprisingly essential for a former football mom like me.

It's a strange thing for me to admit, but I met myself in this circle of Protectors. That is to say, I see myself in them and their relentless need to be strong. I am not the type of human that would spontaneously run into a burning building or race toward the sound of gunfire. I leave that to the able-bodied professionals, unless, of course, my children's lives are at stake. In which case, God help whoever is in my way. Like so many of our nation's Protectors, I am strong to a fault; I always have been. I inherited my mother's indomitable spirit. She had a rough childhood, and so she rarely let down her guard, saving her tears for a rainy day or a hot tub of bubbles behind closed doors at the end of the night. Being vulnerable was never her strong suit, nor is it mine.

God purposefully led me here. I believe that with my whole heart—He knew these courageous men and women who stood (and continue to stand) on the front lines of our country and community needed me to show them love and gratitude and to help them write down their stories. And He knew I needed them, too. These Protectors taught me how to let down my guard with grace. They showed me that it was okay to be vulnerable and to lean on others. And for that, and their trust in me to edit their stories, I will forever be grateful!

Believe me; I know it's not easy handing over one's literary text to be edited, picked apart, assessed, rewritten, corrected, researched, and fact checked. Edit, after all, is a four-letter word! Rehashing someone's written work is akin to taking a weedwhacker to their prized Rhododendrons. It's a wonder any of my clients still send me Christmas cards after I am done. The truth is, writing a book is a lot like giving birth, and I always begin any conversation I have with my prospective clients with this caveat, "This is going to hurt; writing and publishing a book is hard, one of the hardest things you'll ever do, but you have to trust me **and** trust the process."

Mind you, the process is a real bitch, and it (along with your editor) will put you through your paces so to test your mettle, but if you hang in there and you do the work, you will have achieved something most people only ever talk about and for that you can be proud!

*Personally, I like that about the process!*

It's overcoming the hard stuff that makes our lives great—on and off the line. So, to all you Protectors (and football moms) out there, I say, "Your story is your superpower; writing it down and sharing it with others will save lives, beginning with your own."

**God bless America and our Protectors!**

~

### *Connect with Natalie*
*Writer, Serial Editor, Terminal Optimist (For Hire)!*

*Email: girlwriter68@hotmail.com*
*Website: www.nothingbutlovenotes.com*

~

# ABOUT THE AUTHOR

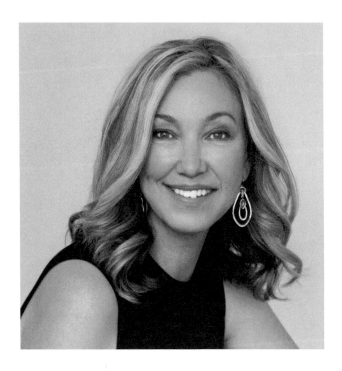

*Sara Correll, Founder The Power of Our Story*

Sara Correll, a dedicated wife and mother of four sons, is passionate about supporting the mental health and transition of our Veterans and First Responders. She created a platform called The Power of Our Story, which holds space for our Protectors to heal, regain hope, and build community through storytelling. As a survivor of suicide loss, Sara intimately understands trauma and the lonely journey of healing. Her advocacy for our Veterans and First Responders was sparked when a US Army Veteran shared his story with her, igniting her passion to help others in similar situations. Through various partnerships and experiences, Sara established "The Power of Our Story: Coffee and Conversation" groups, a safe, judgment-free zone where Veterans and First Responders can share their stories.

Sara holds a Bachelor of Science in Liberal Studies and a certification in drug and alcohol counseling. She is currently pursuing a Master's degree in human services counseling with a focus on crisis response and trauma. Additionally, Sara serves as a coach with The Honor Foundation and as a group facilitator with Waypoint Coaching Inc. Her journey is a testament to her resilience and commitment to making a difference in the lives of those who have sacrificed so much for others. Sara's work continues to inspire and support Protectors on their path to healing and reintegration.

∾

### Connect with Sara
*Founder The Power of Our Story, Counselor and Coach*

*Email: tposleadership@gmail.com*
*Email: Sara@waypointcoachinginc.com*
*LinkedIn: Sara Correll*
*Website: www.thepowerofourstory.com*
*Website: https://waypointcoachinginc.com/*

∾

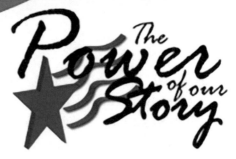

**The Power of our Story**

**Welcomes Veterans, Active-Duty Military, First Responders (active and retired), and Caring Bridge Builders to join us for Coffee & Conversation.**

## PROTECTORS, you have a HOME with us!

Friends, let's process this journey together – We are a tribe of safety to process the journey with others that "get it" – connect with a tribe of Protectors – and a place to find inspiration in a judgment free zone.

**Contact us!**

**Email:** TPOSLeadership@gmail.com
**LinkedIn:** @The Power of Our Story
**Instagram:** @thepowerofourstory
**Facebook:** ThePowerOfOurStory

Made in United States
Troutdale, OR
10/13/2024